PALEO DIET FOR KIDS

SIMPLE GUIDE AND DEDICATED COOKBOOK FOR KIDS TO FOLLOW THE PALEO DIET

By
Jack HARRIS

TABLE OF CONTENS

INTRODUCTION TO PALEO DIET FOR KIDS

BENEFITS OF PALEO DIET

The paleo diet plan is a diet program that mimics how pre-historic people could have eaten. It entails consuming whole food items that people could search for or collect. Promoters from the paleo diet plan decline new diet programs that are usually filled with processed food items. They think that time for how hunter- gatherers consumed could cause fewer health issues. The paleo diet plan isn't safe for everybody. Physicians have no idea of its results on kids, women that are pregnant, or old grownups. Individuals with persistent problems, such as inflammatory intestinal illness, should talk to a physician before trying a paleo diet plan. This manual explores paleo principles, and a 7-day paleo diet meal intends to follow. Please continue reading to understand how to consume like our forefathers. The paleo diet plan's focus is on eating foodstuffs that might have already been obtainable in the Paleolithic era. Furthermore, the paleo diet plan will be referred to as the rock age group diet plan, hunter-gatherer diet plan, or caveman diet plan. Before contemporary agriculture developed around 10,000 years back, people usually ate foods they could hunt or gather, such as fish, liver organs, fruits, vegetables, peanuts, and seeds. The introduction of modern farming changed how people ate. Milk products, dried beans, and grains grew to become a section of people's diet plans. Advocates from the paleo diet plan believe that the body hasn't evolved to procedure dairy products, dried beans, and grains that feed on these food types could raise the threat of specific health issues, such as cardiovascular disease, being overweight, and diabetes.

HEALTH ADVANTAGES OF PALEO

Individuals declare that the paleo diet plan gives numerous health advantages, such as promoting weight reduction, reducing the chance of diabetes, and ecreasing blood pressure. In this area, we go through the scientific evidence to find out what the study facilitates these claims:

EXCESS WEIGHT LOSS

A mature 2008 research discovered that 14 healthy volunteers achieved the average weight reduction of 2.3 kilos by following a paleo diet plan for three weeks. In 2009, researchers compared the paleo diet plan's consequences with the diet plan for diabetes on 13 people with type 2 diabetes. Little research discovered that consuming the paleo method decreased individuals' body weight and waistline area. The 2014 research of 70 post-menopausal ladies with weight problems discovered that carrying out a paleo diet plan helped individuals shed weight after six months. Nevertheless, right after 24 months, there has been simply no difference in weight reduction among individuals following a paleo diet and the ones sticking with regular Nordic nutritional suggestions. These outcomes claim that some other healthy diet programs could be as effective at advertising weight reduction.

The authors of the 2017 review noted that this paleo diet plan helped reduce weight for a while but figured this result is because of caloric restriction or consuming fewer calories. Generally, the study shows that the paleo diet plan can help people shed weight initially, but that additional diet plans that reduce calorie consumption might be effective. Even more, the study is essential before physicians recommend the paleo diet plan for weight reduction. Presently, physicians recommend visitors to follow a calorie- controlled exercise and diet even more to lose excess weight

REDUCING THE RISK OF DIABETES

Does following a Paleo diet program reduce the risk of diabetes? The results of some preliminary research are usually encouraging. Insulin resistance is a dangerous element in the development of diabetes. Improving a person's sensitivity to insulin levels reduces the likelihood that it can lead to diabetes and helps those who have diabetes to reduce their symptoms. A 2015 study compared the consequences of a Paleo diet plan to the consequences of a diet plan predicted by the recommendations of your American Diabetes Association on people who have type 2 diabetes. While both diet programs improved the metabolic health of individuals, the paleo diet

plan improved insulin resistance and blood sugar control. A 2009 study of nine sedentary volunteers without obesity found that the Paleo diet plan improved insulin awareness. There is a requirement for a more recent study for the paleo diet plan and diabetes. However, the evidence to date suggests that a hunter-gatherer-like diet may improve insulin sensitivity.

REDUCING BLOOD PRESSURE

Elevated blood pressure is a prospective factor in cardiovascular disease. Many people believe that a paleo diet plan can help keep blood pressure in balance and promote coronary heart health. Research conducted in 2008 on 14 healthy volunteers found that following a paleo diet plan for 3 weeks improved systolic blood pressure. In addition, overweight and whole-body body mass index (BMI) decreased. The analysis does not add handle to the team, and yet, the results are usually not conclusive. Research from 2014 supported these early results. Experts compared the consequences of a Paleo diet plan with the consequences of a diet plan recommended by Dutch wellness authorities on 34 individuals with traits of metabolic symptoms, a disorder that increases the danger of cardiovascular disease. The outcomes showed how the Paleo diet plan lowered the users' blood pressure and bloodstream lipid profile, which may improve wellness centers. Although preliminary studies claim that the Paleo diet can lower blood pressure and promote heart health, newer and larger studies are needed to draw conclusions.

HOW TO START A DIET

The Paleo diet will supposedly rid you of migraines, eliminate bloating, eliminate seasonal allergies, clear up acne, and shed a few pounds. While none of this is guaranteed, cleaning up your diet and focusing on fresh, wholesome foods is a good idea. Natural foods in reasonable portions will help you feel reasonably satisfied because they help maintain your blood sugar levels.even and hunger hormones completely balanced. Paleo guidelines for beginners:

Sounds simple, however going caveman successfully requires savvy:

SKIP ALL GRAINS

(whole grains and refined), dairy, packaged snacks, legumes and sugar in favor of vegetables, fruits, meats, eggs, seafood, nuts, fats, seeds and oils. For starters, you can follow these paleo diet principles.

PRECISE MOTIVATION

Most individuals turn to the Paleo diet to help with health issues such as gastrointestinal problems, allergies, and autoimmune diseases. Some need to feel good day-to-day or believe it is a healthy way to eat. Your main reason would help you determine the principles to follow and what you need to be careful about. Also, be strict about your guidelines for the very first month. It is a long enough time to start seeing good changes in your health.

CLEAN YOUR KITCHEN

Gather up all the "don't" foods listed on the Paleo diet, such as packaged foods, cereals, milk, cheese, vegetable oils, yogurt, and beans, you got it- and throw them in the trash. Doing all of this has one advantage: it's easy to avoid temptation when it's not there. But if you like to take baby steps at first, then it works just the same. You can probably cut out dairy during the first week, eliminate refined grains during the second week, and cut out grains during the third week, and so on until you're following the Paleo diet. In any case, make sure you buy whole foods; therefore, you have enough to that you can work with to create a Paleo diet meal plan.

FOLLOW THE 85/15 APPROACH

After the 1st 30 days, several experts suggest the 85/15 rule, which means that you stick strictly to the paleo diet 85% of the time and save 15% for non-paleo, whether that's one muesli bar (you could choose this from a paleo muesli recipe), one burger (bun and all) when cooking, or some smoothies. Focus on how you feel after introducing new things to the paleo diet. For example, if you have one scoop of delicious ice cream and wake up bloated the next day, you might decide that the future discomfort isn't worth it

COOK

Because the Paleo diet is based on fresh, whole foods, it's easier to prepare meals at home than at a restaurant, where it's hard to control what ingredients are there. So take advantage of this unique opportunity to experiment with new foods.

You may find it a bit challenging to buy a strange-looking vegetable at the market and ask the vendor for advice on how to prepare it perfectly. You can also search the internet or invest in a paleo diet cookbook for inspiration; that way, the meals will stay tasty and won't just be plain chicken breasts along with simple carrots and kale.

EXPECT 1 FAILURE (OR 2)

It's normal to slip into your usual eating habits when following the Paleo diet. However, you don't have to worry about failure. It's a good learning process. You can also seek out like-minded people who are already following this diet through local forums, groups, blogs, and Facebook and connect with them to take help and keep you on track - and keep you there.

LABEL DECODER

As you know, don't eat doughnuts, crackers and cookies, but a few foods are not paleo: nut butter jars; peanut butter (that's a legume); dried fruit along with added sugars; and lunchmeats, malt vinegar, soy sauce and other sauces and marinades (some consist of sugar, soy, preservatives and gluten). So when buying anything in a packet, make sure you check the list of all ingredients.

THINK ABOUT YOUR PLATE

We teach you to always reserve half your plate for vegetables, a quarter for lean protein, and the remaining quarter for whole grains. As you transition to a Paleo diet, stop saving room for grains. A balanced plate includes a palm-sized protein, one pan of fat, and veggies, veggies, veggies (fill the remaining container along with them).

REPLACE THE OIL

Instead of reaching for corn, canola or soybean oil for frying, you'll need to use lard or coconut oil. Really. Yes, it's good to cook with these good quality saturated fats because they are stable and don't oxidize when cooked (plus oxidation releases harmful free radicals). As for lard, animal fats - in this case from grass-fed cows - have been loaded with huge amounts of omega 3 and one form of fat known as conjugated linoleic acid, which some studies suggest may help you burn fat.

Some dietitians also recommend butter from grass-fed cows; however, many limit dairy products of all kinds. (The choice is yours.) For cold applications, you can use walnut oil, olive oil, and avocado oil.

EAT MEAT

Many people have limited meat in the Paleo diet because they believe it is harmful to health. You can eat meat too - just be sure it's good quality. So you can say goodbye to processed meats, which include salami, hot dogs and sausages.

Wild meats such as bison, boar and elk are excellent choices, followed by pasture-raised poultry as well as meat, and the last choice has to be grain-fed lean meats. And when it comes to seafood, choose wild-caught quite often, with low-mercury and sustainably sourced choices being best.

YOU CAN EASILY FOOL YOUR SWEET TOOTH.

Eliminating sugar is one of the primary difficult tasks for several people in the beginning. In the event that you like to indulge in a treat right after dinner, you can swap cookies or just for yourself for one piece of fruit. (For your sugar cravings, experts say the Paleo diet permits dried mango). Over time, your taste buds would adjust accordingly - and that Oreos you used to love so much may now become so sweet for you. Seriously, it can happen!

YOU CAN EAT OUT

On the paleo diet, it's possible to have a business dinner or brunch with your best friends. All you have to do is do a little digging for ingredients. First, you need to look at the menu beforehand and pick 1 or 2 options that you could paleo modify.

For example, it could be wild salmon and broccoli. (Also, ask for double the vegetables rather than rice pilaf.) Also, don't be shy about asking pertinent questions at the restaurant about what you're preparing and ask for adjustments if necessary.

EAT WHOLESOME, NUTRIENT-DENSE FOODS.If the food is not in the condition it was when it was pulled from the soil, then chances are it has been refined and is not optimal. By choosing foods straight from nature, we provide our bodies with the nutrients that are needed to heal our bodies.

AVOID NUTRIENT-POOR, PROCESSED AND REFINED FOODS THAT ARE PRODUCED IN FACTORIES

This means pasteurized dairy products, grains, seed oils (canola, cottonseed, corn, and soya), artificial sweeteners and refined sugar (high fructose corn syrup). Most of these foods rob the body of nutrients for digestion, which negates the primary goal of diet, which is to fuel the human body and provide it with nutrients for growth and repair. Yes, getting familiar with the paleo lifestyle would take some time. In the beginning, there may be some confusion as you work on changing your habits of grocery shopping, eating out and food preparation; therefore, it is essential to change it at a gradual pace that suits you perfectly. Additionally, know that most "non-paleo" foods need to be reworked to fit the paleo lifestyle.

FOOD FOR A HEALTHY DIGESTIVE SYSTEM

Gut and brain health is extremely important for overall health. To be successful, you need to focus on the signs your body is giving you. In case you find that eating dairy products causes certain digestive problems, then this is your body's way of telling you to avoid these foods! Keeping a food diary and food record could help you discover the latest trends and signs of food consumption. Digestive health is more important than many people think. Did you know that 60 to 80 percent of the immune system starts in the gut? If you were to constantly burden your digestion with certain irritating foods, then your immune system would be suppressed and your health would suffer greatly.

EAT FOODS THAT KEEP BLOOD SUGAR LEVELS STABLE

Have you ever felt weak or shaky between meals? Do you have fluctuations in your energy levels? Chances are your blood sugar levels rise and fall as a result of eating. If you eat sugar and white flour, then your blood sugar levels will spike and you will feel a rush of energy. While the body handles the sugar automatically, the blood sugar level also drops and you start feeling hungry and lethargic. Eating wholesome foods would provide the body with carbohydrates, enough protein and sufficient fats. This combination would allow blood sugar levels to rise even more slowly after meals and remain elevated between meals. Because the Paleo diet is all about eating whole foods, it could be suitable for everyone. The main thing is that it could easily be adapted to suit everyone. Keeping one journal of how you feel throughout the day could make the whole process go smoothly.

Author's note: This book has given you all the information you need to do this diet correctly and do it right. It is essential to understand what you are getting into when you embark on this diet, and this book gave you valuable information that you can use to your advantage and avoid the problems that can come with this diet. You want to stay healthy and make sure that your body can do what it needs to do. As with anything, we emphasize that if something seems wrong or unnatural, you will need to see a doctor to make sure you are safe and that your body can handle this diet. Use the knowledge in this book to get amazing recipes and learn directions for excellent meals for yourself. Consult your doctor before to starting new diet.

BREAKFAST RECIPES

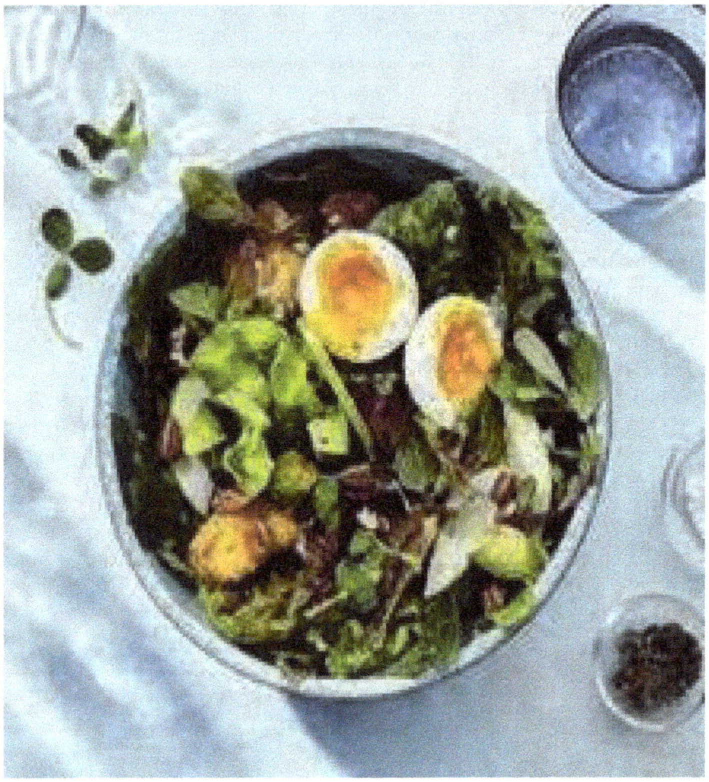

1) MORNING EGG SALAD

Preparation Time: 10 minutes Cooking Time: 0 minutes Servings: 6

Ingredients:

- ½ cup of coconut yogurt
- 4 eggs, hard-boiled
- ½ cup celery stalk, chopped
- 1 tablespoon chives, chopped
- 1 teaspoon chili flakes

Ingredients:

- ½ red onion, chopped
- 2 oz pickles, chopped
- ½ teaspoon salt
- 1 tablespoon fresh dill, chopped

Directions:

- Peel the eggs and chop them.
- Put the chopped eggs in the salad bowl
- Add celery stalk, chives, chili flakes, red onion, and pickles.
- After this, in the separated bowl mix up coconut yogurt, salt, and fresh dill
- Whisk the mixture gently.
- Pour the yogurt mixture over the salad. Mix up the salad well

2) CHICKEN SALAD WITH TAHINI

Preparation Time: 15 minutes Cooking Time: 20 minutes Servings: 4

Ingredients:

- 1 tablespoon tahini sauce
- 1 teaspoon sesame seeds
- 1-pound chicken breast, skinless, boneless
- 1 cup lettuce, chopped

Ingredients:

- ½ teaspoon salt
- 1 teaspoon olive oil
- 1 teaspoon ground black pepper
- 1 tablespoon coconut cream

Directions:

- Chop the chicken breast and mix it up with olive oil, salt, and ground black pepper.
- Put the chicken in the skillet and flatten it in one layer.
- Cook the chicken in the preheated to 365F for 20 minutes.
- Meanwhile, put the chopped lettuce in the salad bowl.

1. Add sesame seeds, salt, and coconut cream.
2. Then add cooked chicken and mix up the salad.
3. Sprinkle the salad with tahini sauce

3) EGG WITH BACON

Preparation Time: 10 minutes | Cooking Time: 17 minutes | Servings: 2

Ingredients:

- 1 teaspoon chives, chopped
- ¼ teaspoon minced garlic
- 2 teaspoons coconut cream
- 2 bacon slices
- 2 eggs, beaten
- 1 teaspoon coconut oil

Directions:

- ❖ Put the coconut oil in the skillet and melt it up on the medium heat.
- ❖ Then place the bacon in the hot oil and cook it for 1 minute from each side.
- ❖ Meanwhile, in the mixing bowl mix up chives, minced garlic, coconut cream, and eggs.
- ❖ Pour the egg mixture over the bacon and close the lid.
- ❖ Cook the meal for 15 minutes over the medium-low heat.

4) GRAIN-FREE NUTTY GRANOLA

Preparation Time: 7 minutes | Cooking Time: 25 minutes | Servings: 6

Ingredients:

- 11/2 cups chopped raw walnuts or pecans 1 cup raw almonds, sliced
- 1/2 cup seeds, toasted or roasted unsalted sunflower, sesame, or shelled pumpkin
- 1/4 cup unsweetened coconut flakes
- 1/2 cup coconut oil or unsalted grass-fed butter, melted 1 tablespoon maple syrup
- 1 teaspoon alcohol-free vanilla extract 1 teaspoon ground cinnamon, or to taste 1/4 teaspoon sea salt or Himalayan salt

Directions:

- ❖ Preheat oven to 300F.
- ❖ Set a rimmed baking sheet with parchment paper or foil.
- ❖ Add the walnuts, almonds, seeds, and coconut flakes to a large bowl
- ❖ In a separate bowl, mix the oil with the maple syrup, vanilla, cinnamon, and salt
- ❖ Pour over the nut mixture, tossing to coat.
- ❖ Scatter the mixture evenly on the prepared baking sheet and bake until golden brown, about 25 minutes
- ❖ Stir once halfway through. Cool completely

5) OVERNIGHT CHIA SEED PUDDING

Preparation Time: 5 minutes Cooking Time: 0 minutes Servings: 1

Ingredients:

- 3 tablespoons chia seeds
- 1 cup coconut milk or unsweetened nut milk
- 1 teaspoon alcohol-free vanilla extract
- 1 teaspoon maple syrup (optional)

Directions:

- In a large jar or bowl, merge all the ingredients, stirring to mix
- Close or cover and refrigerate overnight.
- The next day, add your preferred toppings and enjoy.

6) VEGGIE-EGGY MUFFINS

Preparation Time: 10 minutes Cooking Time: 20 minutes Servings: 6

Ingredients:

- Extra-virgin olive oil, coconut oil, or clarified butter, for greasing (optional)
- 12 large eggs
- 2 teaspoons sea salt or Himalayan salt
- 2 teaspoons freshly ground black pepper 1 medium red bell pepper
- 1 medium orange, yellow, or green bell pepper, seeded and diced 1 cup packed baby spinach, finely chopped
- 1/2 cup thinly sliced scallions
- 1 small jalapeño pepper, seeded and minced (optional)

Directions:

- Preheat the oven to 350F. Grease a 12-hole muffin pan or use paper muffin liners.
- In a large bowl, place the eggs, salt, and pepper and beat until fluffy
- Add the peppers, spinach, scallions, and jalapeño, stirring to combine.
- Ladle the egg mixture evenly into the prepared muffin pan.
- Bake until a toothpick or paring knife comes out clean when inserted, about 20 minutes
- Let the muffins cool before serving.

7) CINNAMON DONUTS

Preparation Time: 20 minutes Cooking Time: 25 minutes Servings: 4

Ingredients:

- 4 tablespoons almond flour
- ½ teaspoon baking soda
- 1 teaspoon lemon juice
- 1 teaspoon ground cinnamon
- 1 egg, beaten
- 1 teaspoon vanilla extract
- 1 tablespoon Erythritol
- 1 tablespoon coconut oil

Directions:

- In the mixing bowl mix up almond flour, baking soda, lemon juice, ground cinnamon, egg, and vanilla extract.
- Knead the soft and non-sticky dough.
- Then roll up the dough.
- Make the donuts with the help of the cutter.
- Line the baking tray with baking paper.
- Then brush it with coconut oil.
- Put the donuts in the tray.
- Cook them for 25 minutes at 365F.
- When the donuts are cooked, sprinkle them with Erythritol.

8) SPINACH MUFFINS

Preparation Time: 10 minutes Cooking Time: 12 minutes Servings: 4

Ingredients:

- 2 cups fresh spinach, chopped
- 4 teaspoons coconut flour
- ½ onion, diced
- 1 teaspoon coconut oil
- ½ teaspoon salt
- ½ teaspoon ground black pepper
- 4 eggs, beaten
- 1 tablespoon coconut cream

Directions:

- Put the spinach in the blender and blend it until smooth.
- Then transfer the spinach in the bowl and add coconut flour, onion, coconut oil, salt,
- Join also ground black pepper, eggs, and coconut cream. Stir the mixture until homogenous.
- After this, pour the mixture in the muffin molds.
- Preheat the oven to 365F.
- Put the muffins in the oven and cook them for 12 minutes

9) TOMATO FRITTATA

Preparation Time: 10 minutes Cooking Time: 17 minutes Servings: 4

Ingredients:

- 1 cup cherry tomatoes, halved
- 1 tablespoon fresh parsley, chopped
- 5 eggs, beaten
- 1 teaspoon coconut oil
- ½ teaspoon salt
- 1/3 teaspoon chili flakes

Directions:

- ❖ In the mixing bowl mix up eggs, salt, and chili flakes,
- ❖ Then place the coconut oil in the skillet and melt it.
- ❖ Put the cherry tomatoes halves in the skillet in one layer
- ❖ Cook them for 1 minute from each side.
- ❖ Then add egg mixture
- ❖ Sprinkle it with fresh parsley and close the lid.
- ❖ Cook the frittata for 15 minutes over the medium heat.

10) EGGS IN ONION RINGS

Preparation Time: 15 minutes Cooking Time: 20 minutes Servings: 2

Ingredients:

- 1 medium onion, peeled
- 2 eggs
- ¼ teaspoon salt
- ¼ teaspoon ground turmeric
- 1 teaspoon almond butter

Directions:

- ❖ Trim the ends of the onion and cut it on 2 slices. Remove the core of the onion slices to get the onion rings.
- ❖ After this, brush the casserole mold with almond butter and put the onion rings inside.
- ❖ Crack the eggs inside the onion rings and sprinkle with salt and ground turmeric.
- ❖ Preheat the oven to 365F.
- ❖ Cover the casserole with eggs with the foil and transfer in the preheated oven.
- ❖ Cook the meal for 20 minutes.

11) BREAKFAST PIZZA

Preparation Time: 10 minutes   Cooking Time: 25 minutes   Servings: 4

Ingredients:

- 4 eggs
- 4 oz ground beef
- 1 cup zucchini, grated
- ½ cup cherry tomatoes, halved
- ¼ cup broccoli, chopped

Ingredients:

- 1 teaspoon ground black pepper
- ¼ teaspoon chili flakes
- ½ teaspoon salt
- 1 teaspoon coconut oil
- 1 teaspoon olive oil

Directions:

- ❖ In the mixing bowl mix up ground beef and zucchini.
- ❖ Then add ground black pepper, chili flakes, and salt.
- ❖ Mix up the mixture and put it in the skillet.
- ❖ Add coconut oil and cook the mixture for 5 minutes.
- ❖ Stir it from time to time.
- ❖ Then add broccoli and mix up the mixture well.
- ❖ Add coconut oil and cook the ground beef mixture for 5 minutes more.
- ❖ Meanwhile, preheat the oven to 365F.
- ❖ Then top the ground beef mixture with cherry tomatoes halves.
- ❖ Crack the eggs over the tomatoes and transfer the skillet in the oven and cook the pizza for 10 minutes

12) CLASSIC SCRAMBLE

Preparation Time: 10 minutes   Cooking Time: 5 minutes   Servings: 3

Ingredients:

- 5 eggs, beaten
- 1 teaspoon olive oil

Ingredients:

- ½ teaspoon salt
- 1 teaspoon white pepper

Directions:

- ❖ Heat up the olive oil in the skillet and add eggs.
- ❖ Cook them for 1 minute and scramble with the help of the fork.
- ❖ After this, sprinkle the scrambled eggs with salt and white pepper and cook for 2 minutes more.
- ❖ Then scramble the eggs again and cook them for 3 minutes.

13) PUMPKIN PANCAKES

Preparation Time: 15 minutes | Cooking Time: 10 minutes | Servings: 6

Ingredients:

- 1 cup pumpkin/butternut squash, grated
- 2 eggs, beaten
- 1 apple, grated
- ½ cup coconut flour
- 1 tablespoon Erythritol
- ½ teaspoon baking powder
- 1 teaspoon ground cinnamon
- 1 teaspoon coconut oil

Directions:

- ❖ In the mixing bowl mix up butternut squash and eggs.
- ❖ Add apple, coconut flour, Erythritol, baking powder, and ground cinnamon. Mix up the mixture well.
- ❖ Then melt the coconut oil in the skillet.
- ❖ Make the pancakes with the help of the spoon in the skillet. Flatten the pancakes if needed.
- ❖ Cook them for 2 minutes from each side over the medium heat.

14) POACHED EGGS IN TOMATO JUICE

Preparation Time: 10 minutes | Cooking Time: 15 minutes | Servings: 4

Ingredients:

- 1 teaspoon garlic, diced
- 1 teaspoon fresh parsley, chopped
- 1 cup tomato juice
- 1 shallot, diced
- 1 teaspoon salt
- 1 teaspoon chili flakes
- 4 eggs
- 1 teaspoon coconut oil

Directions:

- ❖ Pour tomato juice in the pan and bring it to boil.
- ❖ Then add parsley, shallot, salt, chili flakes, and coconut oil.
- ❖ Add garlic and close the lid. Simmer the tomato juice mixture for 5 minutes.
- ❖ After this, crack the eggs over the tomato juice and close the lid.
- ❖ Cook the meal for 10 minutes on the medium heat.

15) ALMOND BUTTER SMOOTHIE

Preparation Time: 5 minutes | Cooking Time: 0 minutes | Servings: 1

Ingredients:

- 1 tablespoon almond butter
- 1 banana, peeled, frozen
- ½ cup blackberries, frozen
- 1 teaspoon raw honey
- ½ cup of coconut milk

Directions:

- ❖ Put the almond butter, banana, blackberries, and coconut milk in the blender.
- ❖ Add raw honey and blend the mixture until smooth
- ❖ Pour the cooked smoothies in the glass.

16) SWEET POTATO HASH

Preparation Time: 10 minutes Cooking Time: 30 minutes Servings: 4

Ingredients:

- 2 sweet potatoes, peeled, chopped
- ½ carrot, chopped
- ½ white onion, chopped
- 1 tablespoon coconut oil
- 3 oz ground beef
- 4 eggs
- ½ teaspoon salt
- ½ teaspoon ground black pepper
- ½ teaspoon ground paprika
- ½ teaspoon dried thyme
- ¼ cup of water

Directions:

- ❖ Put the chopped sweet potatoes in the pan and add coconut oil.
- ❖ Cook the vegetables for 3 minutes.
- ❖ Then stir them well and add carrot, onion, and salt. Mix up well and cook the vegetables for 5 minutes more.
- ❖ After this, add ground beef, ground black pepper, paprika, and thyme. Stir it well.
- ❖ Add water and close the lid.
- ❖ Cook the mixture on the medium heat for 10 minutes.
- ❖ Then open the lid and crack the eggs over the hash.

1. Cook the meal for 10 minutes more

17) GREEN BREAKFAST SMOOTHIE

Preparation Time: 10 minutes Cooking Time: 0 minutes Servings: 2

Ingredients:

- 1/2 Banana, sliced
- 2 cups spinach
- 1 cup sliced berries of your choosing, fresh or frozen
- 1 orange, peeled and cut into segments 1 cup unsweetened nondairy milk
- 1 cup ice

Directions:

- ❖ In a blender, combine all the ingredients.
- ❖ Starting with the blender on low speed, begin blending the smoothie, gradually increasing blender speed until smooth
- ❖ Serve immediately

18) WARM MAPLE AND CINNAMON QUINOA

Preparation Time: 5 minutes | Cooking Time: 15 minutes | Servings: 4

Ingredients:

- 1 cup unsweetened nondairy milk
- 1 cup water
- 1 cup quinoa, rinsed
- 1 teaspoon cinnamon
- 1/4 cup chopped pecans
- 2 tablespoons pure maple syrup or agave

Directions:

- ❖ Bring the almond milk, water, and quinoa to a boil. Lower the heat to medium-low and cover
- ❖ Cook gently until the quinoa softens, about 15 minutes.
- ❖ Turn off the heat and allow sitting, covered, for 5 minutes.
- ❖ Stir in the cinnamon, pecans, and syrup. Serve hot.

19) BLUEBERRY AND CHIA SMOOTHIE

Preparation Time: 10 minutes | Cooking Time: 0 minutes | Servings: 2

Ingredients:

- 2 tablespoons chia seeds
- 2 cups unsweetened nondairy milk 2 cups blueberries, fresh or frozen
- 2 tablespoons pure maple syrup or agave
- 2 tablespoons cocoa powder

Directions:

- ❖ Blend together the soaked chia seeds, almond milk
- ❖ Add blueberries, maple syrup, and cocoa powder and blend until smooth
- ❖ Serve immediately

20) APPLE AND CINNAMON OATMEAL

Preparation Time: 5 minutes | Cooking Time: 15 minutes | Servings: 4

Ingredients:

- 1/4 cups apple cider
- 1 apple, peeled, cored, and chopped
- 2/3 cup rolled oats
- 1 teaspoon ground cinnamon
- 1 tablespoon pure maple syrup

Directions:

- ❖ Take the apple cider to a boil over medium-high heat. Stir in the apple, oats, and cinnamon.
- ❖ Bring the cereal to a boil and turn down heat to low. Simmer until the oatmeal thickens, 3 to 4 minutes
- ❖ Spoon into two bowls and sweeten with maple syrup, if using. Serve hot.

LUNCH RECIPES

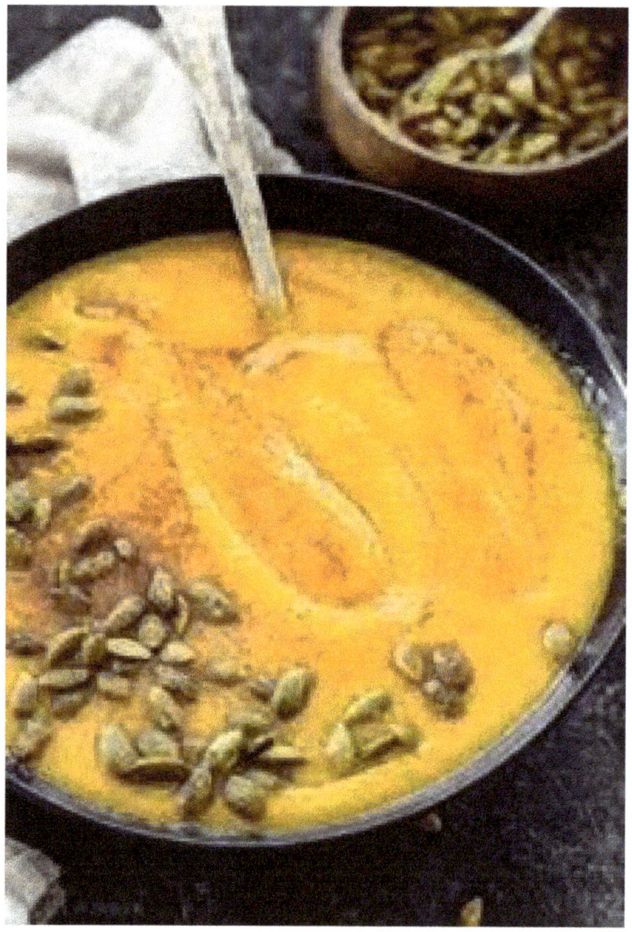

21) ROASTED BUTTERNUT SQUASH PUMPKIN SOUP

Preparation Time: 15 minutes Cooking Time: 40 minutes Servings: 4

Ingredients:

- 2 lbs. butternut squash, peeled chopped into 1-inch pieces
- 1 pumpkin, peeled and chopped
- 1 onion, roughly chopped
- 3 cloves of garlic, minced
- 3 tablespoon olive oil
- 3 sprigs fresh thyme, chopped
- 3 sprigs fresh rosemary chopped
- 1 teaspoon kosher salt
- 1 teaspoon black pepper
- 2 cup low-sodium vegetable broth
- 1/4 cup roasted pumpkin seeds

Directions:

- ❖ Program your oven to 400F, then place the butternut squash, pumpkin, onions, and garlic on a parchment-lined baking sheet
- ❖ Add the olive oil thyme, rosemary, salt, and pepper and toss to coat the ingredients in the seasonings.
- ❖ Roast the pumpkin and butternut squash for 25-35 minutes until it is slightly browned and tender
- ❖ Remove the pumpkin mixture from the oven and allow it to cool slightly.
- ❖ Then a third of the butternut squash mixture to a blender and add about 1/2 cup of the vegetable broth
- ❖ Blend until the soup is smooth
- ❖ Pour the soup into a pot and repeat the process until all of the pumpkin and butternut squash mixture is gone.
- ❖ Heat the roasted butternut squash and pumpkin soup for 4-5 minutes over medium-low heat until the soup is fully heated.
- ❖ Serve and enjoy!

22) SUMMER GAZPACHO

Preparation Time: 25 minutes Cooking Time: 2 hours Servings: 6

Ingredients:

- 3 lbs. ripe red tomatoes, cored and roughly chopped
- 2 cups tomato juice
- 1 sweet yellow onion, roughly chopped into 1-inch pieces
- 1 large cucumber, peeled and seeded
- 1 medium red bell pepper
- ¼ cup fresh basil leaves
- 2 cloves garlic, minced
- 1 tablespoon fresh lemon juice
- ¼ cup extra-virgin olive oil
- 2 tablespoons red wine vinegar
- 1 teaspoon sea salt
- 1/2 teaspoon black pepper

Directions:

- ❖ Add the tomato juice, tomatoes, red pepper, cucumber, onion, basil, garlic
- ❖ Then lemon juice, and olive oil to a blender and blend the vegetables into a smooth puree.
- ❖ Add in the seasonings red wine vinegar, sea salt, black pepper, and blend for an additional 30 seconds.
- ❖ Pour the gazpacho into an airtight container and chill it for 2 hours
- ❖ Before serving, stir the gazpacho to combine the ingredients
- ❖ Pour the gazpacho into six bowls or glasses
- ❖ Garnish with fresh basil, chopped cucumber, and tomatoes, or your preferred toppings.
- ❖ Serve and enjoy!

23) BASIL GARLIC ZUCCHINI NOODLES

Preparation Time: 15 minutes   Cooking Time: 2 minutes   Servings: 4

Ingredients:

- 1 tablespoon olive oil
- 4 spiralized zucchini
- 1 tablespoon freshly chopped basil leaves
- 2 cloves garlic, minced
- 2 tablespoon spinach basil pesto (from the Tomato Red Onion Olive Spinach Pesto Pizza)
- 1 teaspoon kosher salt
- 1/2 teaspoon black pepper
- 1/2 teaspoon red pepper flakes

Directions:

- Place the olive oil into a large skillet over medium-low heat; once it is hot
- Add the garlic and basil and cook for 1 minute until it is aromatic.
- Then in the pesto and the zucchini noodles and sauté for 1-2 minutes
- ❖
- (Until the zucchini noodles are tender).
- Serve and enjoy!

24) MAPLE GLAZED SALMON

Preparation Time: 5 minutes   Cooking Time: 25 minutes   Servings: 4

Ingredients:

- 1/3 cup maple syrup
- 1/4 coconut aminos
- 2 tablespoon lemon juice
- 1 tablespoon orange juice
- 1 teaspoon red pepper flakes
- 3 tablespoon extra-virgin avocado oil, divided
- 4 6-oz. salmon fillets
- 1 teaspoon sea salt
- 1/2 teaspoon black pepper
- 3 cloves garlic, minced
- 1 teaspoon ginger, minced

Directions:

- Whisk the maple syrup, coconut aminos, lemon juice, orange juice and red pepper flakes in a medium bowl.
- Pat your salmon filets dry using a paper towel
- Place two tablespoons of avocado oil into a large skillet set over medium-high heat
- Once the avocado oil is hot, place the salmon skin-side up into the pan
- Season with the sea salt and black pepper
- Sear the salmon for 5-6 minutes until it is a rich golden brown color
- Cook salmon until deeply golden.
- Turn the maple glazed salmon over and add the remaining tablespoon of avocado oil
- Add minced garlic and ginger to the salmon and cook for 1 minute until aromatic.
- Then he maple syrup mixture, decrease the heat to medium-low and cook the salmon until sauce is reduced by 1/3
- Brush the salmon with the maple sauce. Serve and enjoy!

25) HERB ROASTED VEGETABLE MEDLEY

Preparation Time: 5 minutes   Cooking Time: 25 minutes   Servings: 6

Ingredients:

- 3 tablespoons olive oil
- 1 teaspoon freshly chopped basil leaves
- 1 teaspoon dried thyme
- 1 teaspoon fresh rosemary
- 2 cloves garlic, minced
- 1 teaspoon salt
- 1⁄2 teaspoon black pepper
- 1 red onion, sliced

Ingredients:

- 1 red bell pepper, sliced
- 1 yellow bell pepper
- 1 green bell pepper
- 2 eggplant, sliced lengthwise and cut into 1/2-inch slices
- 4 medium zucchini, cut into 1/2-inch slices
- 1 large carrot, cut into 1/2-inch slices

Directions:

- ❖ Program the oven to 450F, then line a baking sheet with parchment paper
- ❖ Add the olive oil, basil, thyme, rosemary, garlic, salt, and pepper to a large bowl and stir to combine.
- ❖ Then the onion, bell peppers, eggplant, zucchini, and carrot and toss to coat the vegetables in the herbs and oil.
- ❖ Arrange the seasoned vegetables on the prepared baking sheet and roast them in the oven for 30 minutes.
- ❖ Serve and enjoy!

26) ROASTED SPAGHETTI SQUASH WITH MARINA SAUCE

Preparation Time: 15 minutes   Cooking Time: 55 minutes   Servings: 8

Ingredients:

- 1 4 lb. spaghetti squash
- 4 tablespoons olive oil
- 1 teaspoon salt
- 1/2 teaspoon black pepper

Ingredients:

- 1 yellow onion, minced
- 2 cloves garlic, minced
- 2 tablespoons fresh basil
- 3 cups marinara sauce

Directions:

- ❖ Program the oven to 375F degrees, then cut the spaghetti squash in half lengthwise, remove the seeds and excess fibers
- ❖ Brush two tablespoons of olive oil onto the spaghetti squash's flesh and place it skin side up onto a parchment- lined cookie sheet.
- ❖ Roast the spaghetti squash for 30-45 minutes until the flesh is soft and tender
- ❖ Remove the squash from the oven and set it aside.
- ❖ Place the remaining two tablespoons of the olive oil in a saucepot set over medium-high heat
- ❖ Then add the minced onions and sauté for 3-4 minutes until they soften, then stir in the garlic and basil and cook for 1 minute until aromatic
- ❖ Add the marinara sauce and cook for 3-4 minutes until the sauce is heated through.
- ❖ Use a fork to scrape the spaghetti squash's strands from the inside of the squash
- ❖ Place the spaghetti squash strands onto your serving dishes and top with the marinara sauce
- ❖ Serve and enjoy!

27) QUINOA TABBOULEH

Preparation Time: 15 minutes Cooking Time: 15 minutes Servings: 4

Ingredients:

- 1 cup quinoa, rinsed well
- 1/2 cup water
- 3/4 cup low-sodium vegetable broth
- 2 teaspoon kosher salt
- 4 tablespoon fresh lemon juice
- 2 garlic clove, minced
- 1/2 cup extra-virgin olive oil

Ingredients:

- 1/2 teaspoon black pepper
- 1 large English cucumber cut into 1/4» pieces
- 1 cup cherry tomatoes halved
- 1/2 cup chopped flat-leaf parsley
- 1/4 cup chopped fresh mint
- 3 scallions, thinly sliced

Directions:

- ❖ Add the quinoa, 1 teaspoon salt, water, and vegetable broth to a medium saucepan over medium-high heat
- ❖ Bring the quinoa to a boil, decrease the heat to medium-low, cover the pot with the lid, and cook the quinoa for 10 minutes until it is tender
- ❖ Take the quinoa off of the stove and let it rest for 5 minutes covered before fluffing with a fork.
- ❖ Meantime, place the lemon juice and garlic into a small bowl, whisk to combine, then slowly whisk in olive oil.
- ❖ Season the dressing with the remaining kosher salt and pepper.
- ❖ Pour the quinoa onto a large sheet pan and spread it into an even layer to cool
- ❖ Once the quinoa is thoroughly cooled, place it into a large bowl
- ❖ Add about 1/3 cup of the tabouleh dressing and mix to combine.
- ❖ Stir in the cucumber, tomatoes, parsley, mint, and scallions
- ❖ Stir to combine, and pour over the remaining dressing
- ❖ Serve and enjoy!

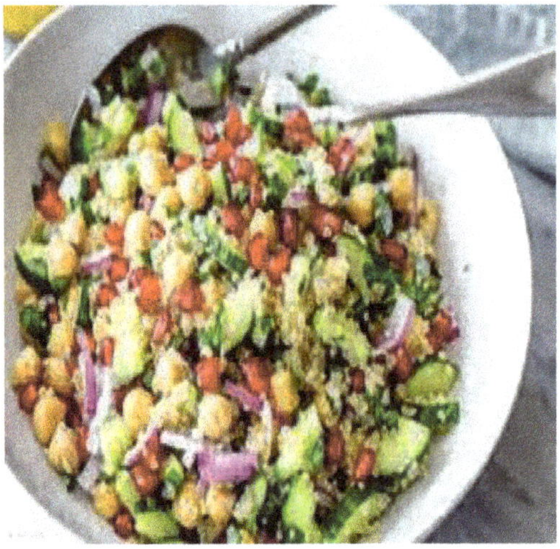

28) STIR-FRY BULGOGI EGGPLANT

Preparation Time: 15 minutes Cooking Time: 15 minutes Servings: 4

Ingredients:

- 1 small onion, minced
- 3 garlic cloves, minced
- 1 scallion, finely chopped
- 2 tablespoon agave nectar
- 1 tablespoon coconut aminos
- 2 teaspoon red pepper flakes
- 1 teaspoon toasted sesame oil
- 1 tablespoon kosher salt
- 1 lb. eggplants
- 1 tablespoon olive oil

Directions:

- ❖ Add the onion, garlic, scallion, agave nectar, coconut aminos, red pepper flakes, and sesame oil to a medium bowl and whisk to combine.
- ❖ Slice the eggplants in half crosswise, then cut the eggplant into 1/4-inch strips
- ❖ Cut the 1/2 inch strips into 1/2 inch wide strips, then place the eggplant in a large bowl with the kosher salt
- ❖ Stir until every piece of eggplant is coated with salt crystals and let it sit for 15-20 minutes, stirring at 5-minute intervals.
- ❖ Drain the liquid from the eggplant, then use your hands to squeeze the las much of the liquid from the eggplant as you can
- ❖ Place the eggplant into a clean bowl, pour the marinade over the eggplant, and toss to combine
- ❖ Cover the bulgogi eggplant with plastic wrap and place it in the refrigerator for 30 minutes.
- ❖ Place the olive oil into a large skillet over high heat and add the eggplant in an even layer once it is hot
- ❖ Sear the eggplant fr 2-3 minutes until the bottom is slightly brown
- ❖ Flip the eggplant and let the other side cook for 2-3 minutes until it is browned
- ❖ Lower the flame to medium-low
- ❖ Cook the eggplant for 5-6 minutes, flipping every so often until the eggplant is completely cooked
- ❖ Serve and enjoy!

29) CREAMY CHICKPEA CURRY

Preparation Time:5 minutes Cooking Time: 30 minutes Servings: 4

Ingredients:

- 2 tablespoon avocado oil
- 1 red onion, chopped
- 2 cloves garlic, crushed
- 1 large tomato, diced
- 1 small carrot thinly sliced into strips
- 1 tablespoon garam masala
- 2 tablespoon red curry paste
- 1/2 teaspoon ground cumin
- 1/2 teaspoon, ground coriander
- 1/4 teaspoon cayenne pepper
- 2 15oz. cans chickpeas, drained
- 1 14oz. can unsweetened coconut milk
- 1 teaspoon kosher salt
- 1/2 teaspoon black pepper

Directions:

- ❖ Place the olive oil into a heavy bottom saucepot
- ❖ Once it is hot, add the red onions, garlic, garam masala, cumin, coriander powder
- ❖ Then cayenne pepper and sauté until the onions soften.
- ❖ Add the chopped tomatoes and sauté for 3-4 minutes until the tomatoes have cooked down
- ❖ Stir in the chickpeas, chopped carrots, and coconut milk, then bring the chickpea curry to a simmer
- ❖ Let the curry simmer for 8-10 minutes
- ❖ Then add the salt and black pepper. Serve and enjoy!

30) SPAGHETTI SQUASH CASSEROLE

Preparation Time: 10 minutes | Cooking Time: 40 minutes | Servings: 6

Ingredients:

- 1-pound chicken breast
- 10 oz spaghetti squash, peeled
- 1 cup cauliflower, chopped, cooked
- 1 teaspoon salt
- 1 teaspoon chili powder
- 1 teaspoon onion powder
- 1 tablespoon coconut oil
- 1 teaspoon olive oil
- 1 teaspoon dried rosemary
- ½ cup coconut cream

Directions:

- Chop the spaghetti squash into tiny pieces.
- Then chop the chicken on the same pieces as spaghetti squash.
- After this, transfer the spaghetti squash in the bowl and add salt, chili powder, onion powder, and dried rosemary.
- Mix up well.
- After this, mix up chopped chicken breast and olive oil.
- Grease the casserole mold with coconut oil and put the chicken inside in one layer.
- Then top it with chopped spaghetti squash mixture, cauliflower, and spread with coconut cream.
- Cover the casserole with foil and secure the edges of the mold.
- Preheat the oven to 375F.
- Put the casserole in the oven and cook it for 40 minutes.

31) VEAL SOUP

Preparation Time: 10 minutes | Cooking Time: 30 minutes | Servings: 4

Ingredients:

- 1-pound veal meat
- 4 cups beef broth
- 3 oz celery root, chopped
- 1 teaspoon dried rosemary
- ½ teaspoon ground cumin
- ½ teaspoon salt
- 1 eggplant, chopped
- 1 teaspoon almond butter

Directions:

- Cu the veal meat on the small cubes and sprinkle them with dried rosemary, ground cumin, and salt.
- Put the almond butter in the saucepan and melt it.
- Add veal cubes and roast them for 5 minutes. Stir the meat from time to time.
- After this, add celery root, eggplant, and beef broth.
- Close the lid and cook the soup for 25 minutes over the medium heat or until the veal is soft.

32) CARROT POTAGE

Preparation Time: 15 minutes | Cooking Time: 45 minutes | Servings: 4

Ingredients:

- 1 cup carrot, chopped
- ½ cup turnip, chopped
- 1 sweet potato, chopped
- ½ yellow onion, diced
- 1 teaspoon coconut oil
- • ½ teaspoon ground black pepper
- 1 teaspoon salt
- 1 teaspoon chives, chopped
- 1 bay leaf
- 1 teaspoon garlic, diced
- ½ teaspoon dried thyme
- 1 cup of water

Directions:

- ❖ Put onion, ground black pepper, salt, bay leaf, garlic, and dried thyme in the saucepan.
- ❖ Add coconut oil and cook the ingredients for 5 minutes over the medium heat. Stir them from time to time with the help of the spatula.
- ❖ Then add water, carrot, turnip, and sweet potato.
- ❖ Close the lid and cook the meal for 40 minutes over the medium heat.
- ❖ When the time is over, remove the bay leaf from the mixture.
- ❖ Blend the vegetable mixture in the food processor until smooth and ladle in the bowls.
- ❖ Top the carrot potage with chives.

33) CREAM OF BROCCOLI SOUP

Preparation Time: 15 minutes | Cooking Time: 30 minutes | Servings: 2

Ingredients:

- 3 cups broccoli, chopped
- 4 cups vegetable stock
- 1 teaspoon minced garlic
- 1 teaspoon salt
- ½ teaspoon ground ginger

Directions:

- ❖ Put broccoli, vegetable stock, minced garlic, salt, and ground ginger in the saucepan.
- ❖ Close the lid and cook the ingredients for 30 minutes.
- ❖ 3. Then transfer it in the food processor and blend until you get a creamy texture.
- ❖ Transfer the cream soup in the saucepan and bring it to boil.
- ❖ Ladle the cooked soup in the serving bowls.

34) BEEF AND CARROT STEW

Preparation Time: 10 minutes | Cooking Time: 65 minutes | Servings: 4

Ingredients:

- 1-pound beef shank, boneless, chopped
- 2 carrots, roughly chopped
- 1 bay leaf
- 1 teaspoon peppercorn
- 2 cups vegetable stock
- 1 teaspoon salt
- 1 white onion, roughly chopped
- 1 teaspoon olive oil

Directions:

- ❖ Pour olive oil in the saucepan and heat it up.
- ❖ Add beef shank and cook it for 2 minutes from each side.
- ❖ Then add roughly chopped carrot, bay leaf, peppercorns, salt, onion, and vegetable stock.
- ❖ Close the lid and cook the stew for 60 minutes over the medium heat.

35) HAM CHOWDER

Preparation Time: 10 minutes | Cooking Time: 30 minutes | Servings: 4

Ingredients:

- 7 oz ham, chopped
- 3 celery stalks, chopped
- ½ green onion, chopped
- ¼ teaspoon garlic powder
- ½ carrot, grated
- ½ cup turnip, chopped
- 3 cups chicken stock
- 1 teaspoon coconut oil
- 1 teaspoon salt
- ½ teaspoon dried rosemary
- 1/3 teaspoon chili flakes

Directions:

- ❖ Put the coconut oil in the saucepan and melt it.
- ❖ Then add grated carrot and green onion.
- ❖ Roast the vegetables for 5 minutes. Stir them from time to time to avoid burning.
- ❖ Then add celery stalk, turnip, garlic powder, salt, rosemary, and chili flakes. Stir the ingredients well and add chicken stock.
- ❖ Bring the mixture to boil and simmer for 10 minutes.
- ❖ Then add chopped ham and cook the soup for 15 minutes more.

36) BISON STEW

Preparation Time: 20 minutes | Cooking Time: 25 minutes | Servings: 4

Ingredients:

- 1-pound ground bison
- 3 oz rutabaga, chopped
- ½ cup kale, chopped
- 2 cups vegetable stock
- ½ cup Brussel sprouts, roughly chopped
- 1 teaspoon smoked paprika
- ½ teaspoon salt
- ½ teaspoon ground cumin
- ¼ teaspoon dried thyme
- 1 teaspoon cayenne pepper

Directions:

- ❖ In the mixing bowl mix up ground bison, smoked paprika, salt, ground cumin, dried thyme, and cayenne pepper.
- ❖ Then put the meat mixture in the pan.
- ❖ Add vegetable stock and bring the mixture to boil. Cook it for 5 minutes more.
- ❖ After this, add rutabaga, Brussel sprouts, and simmer the stew for 10 minutes over the medium heat.
- ❖ When the Brussel sprouts are soft, add kale and cook the stew for 10 minutes on the low heat.
- ❖ Let the cooked stew rest for 20 minutes.

37) CRAB STEW

Preparation Time: 10 minutes | Cooking Time: 15 minutes | Servings: 3

Ingredients:

- 14 oz crab meat, chopped
- 2 shallots, chopped
- 1 jalapeno pepper, sliced
- 1 tomato, chopped
- ¼ cup tomato juice
- 1 teaspoon cumin seeds
- ¼ teaspoon fennel seeds
- 1 cup fish stock

Directions:

- ❖ Put shallots in the saucepan.
- ❖ Add jalapeno pepper, cumin seeds, fennel seeds, and fish stock.
- ❖ Add tomato and tomato juice.
- ❖ Bring the mixture to boil and simmer it for 5 minutes.
- ❖ Then add chopped crab meat and cook the stew on the low heat for 10 minutes.
- ❖ Let the cooked stew rest for 10 minutes before serving.

38) VEG&MEAT STEW

Preparation Time: 10 minutes | Cooking Time: 55 minutes | Servings: 2

Ingredients:

- 4 oz asparagus, chopped
- 4 oz broccoli, chopped
- 10 oz beef shank, chopped
- 1 cup chicken stock
- ½ teaspoon peppercorn
- 1 bay leaf
- 1 teaspoon salt
- 1 teaspoon tapioca flour

Directions:

- Pour the chicken stock in the pan.
- Add beef shank, peppercorns, bay leaf, and salt.
- Then close the lid and cook the meat mixture for 40 minutes on the medium heat.
- After this, add asparagus and broccoli.
- Cook the stew for 10 minutes more.
- Add tapioca flour and stir the stew until flour is dissolved.
- Cook the stew for 5 minutes more. All the ingredients of the stew should be very soft.

39) PORK CHOPS WITH ZUCCHINI NOODLES

Preparation Time: 15 minutes | Cooking Time: 20 minutes | Servings: 2

Ingredients:

- 2 pork chops
- 1 zucchini, trimmed
- ½ teaspoon smoked paprika
- ½ teaspoon salt
- ½ teaspoon cayenne pepper
- 2 teaspoons olive oil
- ¼ cup of coconut milk
- ½ cup chicken stock

Directions:

- Rub the pork chops with smoked paprika, salt, and cayenne pepper.
- Then brush them with olive oil and put in the skillet.
- Cook the pork chops for 5 minutes from each side.
- After this, pour the chicken stock in the saucepan and bring it to boil.
- Make the noodles from the zucchini with the help of the spiralizer and put in the hot chicken stock. Boil the noodles for 3 minutes and transfer them in the serving bowls.
- Then add the cooked pork chops in the chicken stock and boil them for 5 minutes.
- Add the pork chops in the zucchini noodles bowls and sprinkle with chicken stock.

40) IRISH STEW

Preparation Time: 10 minutes Cooking Time: 55 minutes Servings: 4

Ingredients:

- 1-pound beef stew meat, chopped
- 1 yellow onion, chopped
- 1 carrot, chopped
- 2 oz parsnip, chopped
- 1 tablespoon sunflower oil
- 1 teaspoon salt
- 2 cups vegetable broth
- 1 tablespoon lemon juice
- ½ cup white cabbage, sliced
- 1 teaspoon minced garlic
- 1 teaspoon raw honey
- ½ teaspoon dried cilantro

Directions:

- Put the chopped beef stew meat in the pan and add vegetable broth.
- Bring the meat to boil and cook it for 15 minutes over the medium heat.
- Meanwhile, in the mixing bowl mix up salt and dried cilantro. Add the spices in the boiling meat. Keep cooking the meat.
- Then pour oil in the skillet and heat it up.
- Add chopped onion and fry it until it is light brown.
- Add the onion in the boiling meat.
- Then add chopped carrot, parsnip, white cabbage, honey, and minced garlic.
- Add lemon juice and close the lid.
- Preheat the oven to 365F.
- Put the pan with the stew in the preheated oven and cook it for 40 minutes.

SNACK RECIPES

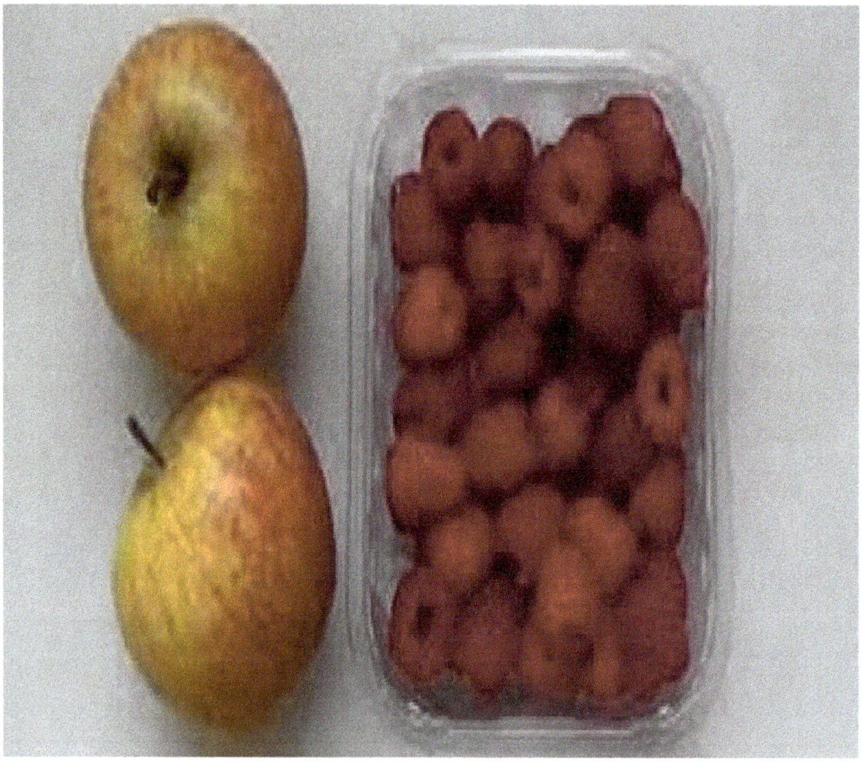

41) GRILLED PEACHES

Preparation Time: 10 minutes | Cooking Time: 2 minutes | Servings: 4

Ingredients:

- 4 peaches, pitted
- ¼ teaspoon almond butter
- 1 teaspoon raw honey

Directions:

- ❖ Preheat the grill to 375F.
- ❖ Cut the peaches into halves.
- ❖ Then sprinkle the peaches with almond butter and put in the grill.
- ❖ Cook them for 1 minute from each side.
- ❖ Sprinkle the cooked peaches with raw honey.

42) RASPBERRY AND APPLE FRUIT LEATHER

Preparation Time: 10 minutes | Cooking Time: 45 minutes | Servings: 6

Ingredients:

- 1 cup raspberries
- ½ cup apple, chopped

Directions:

- ❖ Preheat the oven to 345F.
- ❖ Line the baking tray with baking paper.
- ❖ After this, put the raspberries and apples in the blender and blend until you get a smooth mixture.
- ❖ Pour it in the baking tray and flatten well.
- ❖ Bake the mixture for 45 minutes or until it is dry.
- ❖ Then cut it into strips and roll into rolls.

43) BAKED APPLE WITH HAZELNUTS

Preparation Time: 15 minutes | Cooking Time: 20 minutes | Servings: 8

Ingredients:

- 4 Granny Smith apples
- 4 teaspoons almond butter
- 2 tablespoons raw honey
- 2 oz hazelnuts, chopped

Directions:

- ❖ Cut the apples into halves and remove seeds.
- ❖ Then make the medium size holes in the apple halves
- ❖ Fill them with almond butter, raw honey, and hazelnuts.
- ❖ Place the apples in the tray and bake for 20 minutes at 350F.

44) CHOCOLATE ENERGY BALLS

Preparation Time: 15 minutes | Cooking Time: 0 minutes | Servings: 5

Ingredients:

- 4 dates, chopped
- 3 oz cashew, chopped
- 1 tablespoon cocoa powder

Directions:

- Put the dates in the blender and blend until you get a smooth mixture.
- Then add cashew and cocoa powder.
- Blend mixture for 30 seconds more.
- Then remove it from the blender and make 5 energy balls with the help of the fingertips.

45) TURKEY STICKS

Preparation Time: 15 minutes | Cooking Time: 0 minutes | Servings: 4

Ingredients:

- 6 oz turkey breast, skinless, boneless
- 1 teaspoon tomato paste
- ½ teaspoon ground turmeric
- 1 tablespoon olive oil
- ½ teaspoon lemon juice

Directions:

- Cut the turkey breast on medium-size sticks (strips).
- Then mix up together tomato paste and olive oil.
- Add lemon juice and ground turmeric.
- After this, mix up turkey sticks and oil mixture.
- Preheat the skillet until it is hot.
- Put the turkey sticks in the skillet in one layer and roast them for 5 minutes from each side or until they turkey sticks are a little bit crunchy.

46) VEGGIE STICKS

Preparation Time: 10 minutes | Cooking Time: 0 minutes | Servings: 4

Ingredients:

- 1 red sweet pepper
- 2 celery stalks
- 1 carrot, peeled
- 1 teaspoon coconut cream
- ¼ teaspoon tahini paste

Directions:

- Cut the sweet pepper, celery stalk, and carrot into the sticks.
- Then put them in the plate side-by-side and sprinkle with coconut cream and tahini paste.

47) PLANTAIN CHIPS

Preparation Time: 10 minutes | Cooking Time: 60 minutes | Servings: 4

Ingredients:

- 2 plantains

Directions:

- Line the baking tray with baking paper.
- Then slice the plantains into the chips slices.
- Put them on the tray in one layer.
- Bake the chips for 60 minutes at 340F.

48) ZUCCHINI HUMMUS

Preparation Time: 10 minutes | Cooking Time: 0 minutes | Servings: 5

Ingredients:

- 2 zucchinis, chopped
- 1 garlic clove, diced
- 1 tablespoon tahini paste

Ingredients:

- 3 tablespoons olive oil
- 1 teaspoon harissa

Directions:

- Put the chopped zucchini in the blender.
- Add garlic, tahini paste, olive oil, and harissa.
- Blend the mixture until smooth.
- Transfer the cooked smooth hummus in the serving bowl.

49) STUFFED MUSHROOM CAPS

Preparation Time: 15 minutes | Cooking Time: 30 minutes | Servings: 4

Ingredients:

- 2 cups mushroom caps
- 1 cup ground chicken
- 1 tablespoon fresh parsley, chopped

Ingredients:

- 1 teaspoon minced garlic
- 1 teaspoon olive oil
- ½ teaspoon salt

Directions:

- Trim the mushroom caps if needed.
- After this, in the mixing bowl mix up ground chicken, parsley, minced garlic, and salt.
- Fill the mushroom caps with ground chicken mixture.
- Then sprinkle them with olive oil and transfer in the baking mold.
- Bake the mushroom caps for 30 minutes at 350F.

50) AVOCADO SALSA

Preparation Time: 5 minutes | Cooking Time: 0 minutes | Servings: 6

Ingredients:

- 1 avocado, chopped
- 1 red onion, chopped
- 2 tomatoes, chopped
- 2 tablespoons fresh cilantro, chopped
- 1 chili pepper, chopped
- 1 tablespoon olive oil
- ½ teaspoon salt
- 1 teaspoon lime juice

Directions:

- ❖ In the mixing bowl mix up red onion, tomatoes, cilantro, chili pepper, olive oil, salt, and lime juice.
- ❖ Then add avocado and stir the cooked salsa well.

51) PARMA MELON

Preparation Time: 15 minutes | Cooking Time: 0 minutes | Servings: 6

Ingredients:

- 1-pound melon
- 4 oz parma ham, sliced

Directions:

- ❖ Peel the melon and cut it on the medium size cubes.
- ❖ Then wrap every melon cube in the parma ham and secure with the toothpick.

52) BABA GHANOUSH

Preparation Time: 15 minutes | Cooking Time: 30 minutes | Servings: 5

Ingredients:

- 2 eggplants
- 1 teaspoon ground cumin
- 1 garlic clove, diced
- 1 tablespoon fresh cilantro
- ½ teaspoon salt
- 1 tablespoon sesame oil
- 1 teaspoon tahini paste

Directions:

- ❖ Pierce the eggplants with the help of the fork and put on the tray.
- ❖ Bake the vegetables for 30 minutes at 365F or until they are soft.
- ❖ Then cool the eggplants gently and peel.
- ❖ Chop the peeled eggplants and put them in the blender.
- ❖ Add diced garlic, ground cumin, fresh cilantro, salt, sesame oil, and tahini paste.
- ❖ Blend the mixture until it is smooth.
- ❖ Transfer the cooked baba ghanoush in the bowl

53) SWEET PEPPER HUMMUS

Preparation Time: 25 minutes | Cooking Time: 25 minutes | Servings: 6

Ingredients:

- 1 teaspoon tahini paste
- 3 tablespoon sesame oil
- ½ teaspoon salt
- 1 cup pumpkin, chopped
- 2 sweet peppers, chopped
- 1 teaspoon olive oil
- ½ teaspoon ground black pepper
- 1 garlic clove, peeled
- 4 tablespoons lemon juice

Directions:

- ❖ Put the pumpkin and sweet pepper in the tray and sprinkle with olive oil.
- ❖ Bake the vegetables for 25 minutes at 375F.
- ❖ Then transfer them in the food processor.
- ❖ Add sesame oil, salt, ground black pepper, garlic clove, and lemon juice.
- ❖ Blend the mixture until it is smooth.
- ❖ Transfer the cooked hummus in the serving bowl.

54) GUACAMOLE

Preparation Time: 15 minutes | Cooking Time: 0 minutes | Servings: 5

Ingredients:

- 1 avocado, pitted, peeled
- 1 garlic clove, diced
- 1 jalapeno pepper, chopped
- 3 oz red onion, diced
- 1 tomato, chopped
- 4 tablespoons lemon juice
- 1 tablespoon fresh cilantro, chopped
- ¼ teaspoon salt
- ½ teaspoon ground black pepper

Directions:

- ❖ Put the garlic clove, jalapeno pepper, red onion, tomato, and fresh cilantro in the mixing bowl.
- ❖ Stir the ingredients until you get a homogenous mixture.
- ❖ After this, mash avocado with salt, ground black pepper, and lemon juice.
- ❖ Add the mashed avocado in the mixing bowl.
- ❖ Mix up guacamole until you get the homogenous texture.

55) CAULIFLOWER POPCORN

Preparation Time: 10 minutes Cooking Time: 15 minutes Servings: 3

Ingredients:

- 1 cup cauliflower florets
- 1 tablespoon coconut oil, melted
- ½ teaspoon salt
- ½ teaspoon ground paprika
- ½ teaspoon ground turmeric
- ½ teaspoon chili flakes
- ¼ cup coconut flour
- 1 tablespoon water

Directions:

- ❖ In the mixing bowl mix up melted coconut oil, salt
- ❖ Add ground paprika, turmeric, chili flakes, and water.
- ❖ Then sprinkle the cauliflower florets with coconut oil mixture well.
- ❖ After this, coat every cauliflower floret in the coconut flour.
- ❖ Arrange the cauliflower in the tray in one layer
- ❖ Cook in the preheated to 360F oven for 15 minutes or until the cauliflower is light brown.

56) TRAIL MIX

Preparation Time: 10 minutes Cooking Time: 5 minutes Servings: 3

Ingredients:

- 3 tablespoons almond flakes
- 3 tablespoons pumpkin seeds
- 1 tablespoon coconut shred
- 3 tablespoons sunflower seeds

Directions:

- ❖ Preheat the skillet until hot.
- ❖ Then put all ingredients from the list above in the hot skillet and mix up.
- ❖ Close the lid and leave the mixture for 10 minutes.

57) ENERGY BALLS

Preparation Time: 15 minutes Cooking Time: 0 minutes Servings: 6

Ingredients:

- 5 oz dates, chopped
- ¼ cup coconut flour
- 1/3 cup almond flour
- 1 tablespoon coconut shred
- 1 tablespoon raw honey

Directions:

- ❖ Put the dates in the blender.
- ❖ Add coconut flour, coconut shred, almond flour, and raw honey.
- ❖ Blend the mixture until it is smooth.
- ❖ Then make the balls from the date smooth mixture
- ❖ Make it with the help of the fingertips.

58) ALMOND CRACKERS

Preparation Time: 20 minutes | Cooking Time: 12 minutes | Servings: 8

Ingredients:

- 6 oz almond flour
- 1 egg, beaten
- ¼ teaspoon ground cumin
- ½ teaspoon salt

Directions:

- In the mixing bowl mix up almond flour, egg, ground cumin, and salt.
- Knead the dough.
- After this, roll it up and cut it into the squares (cracker shapes).
- Line the baking tray with the baking paper and put the uncooked crackers inside.
- Cook the crackers at 360F for 12 minutes or until the edges of the crackers are light brown

59) AVOCADO FRIES

Preparation Time: 10 minutes | Cooking Time: 5 minutes | Servings: 4

Ingredients:

- 1 avocado, pitted
- 2 eggs, beaten
- ¼ cup coconut shred
- 1 tablespoon olive oil

Directions:

- Cut the avocado on 4 wedges and then peel every avocado wedge.
- Pour olive oil in the skillet and heat it up.
- Meanwhile, dip the avocado wedges in the beaten eggs and then coat in the coconut shred.
- Repeat step 3 one more time.
- Then place the avocado wedges in the hot olive oil
- Cook them for 1 minute from each side on the medium heat

60) CABBAGE CHIPS

Preparation Time: 15 minutes | Cooking Time: 17 minutes | Servings: 6

Ingredients:

- 1-pound savoy cabbage
- 1 teaspoon sesame seeds
- 1 teaspoon ground cumin
- 1 teaspoon dried basil
- 2 tablespoons olive oil
- ½ teaspoon salt

Directions:

- 1. Separate the savoy cabbage on the leaves and then cut into the small petals (chips).
- 2. Line the baking tray with baking paper.
- 3. Put the savoy cabbage petals in the tray and flatten them in one layer.
- 4. Sprinkle the vegetables with sesame seeds, cumin, basil, olive oil, and salt.
- 5. Cook the cabbage chips in the preheated to 155F oven for 17 minutes.
- 6. Shake the cabbage chips during cooking from time to time.

DINNER RECIPES

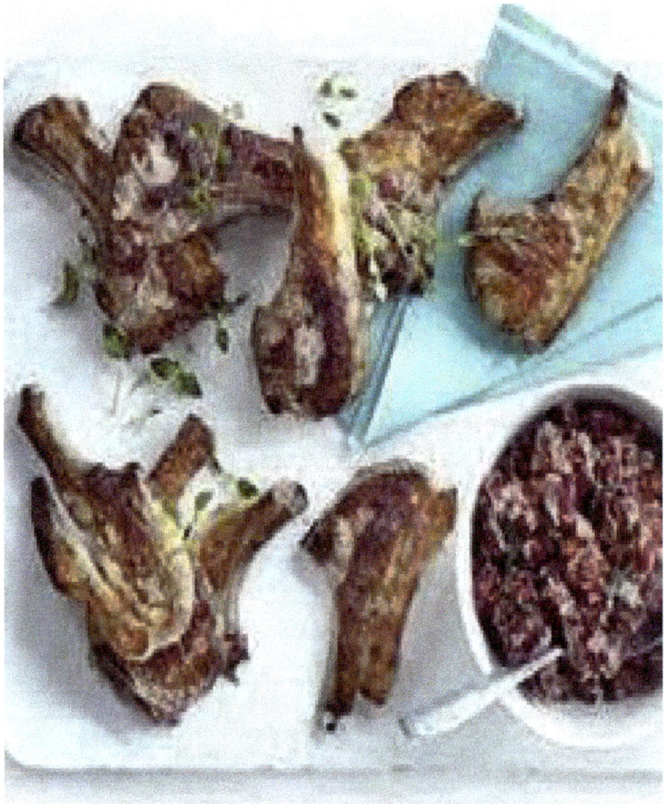

61) SUPER TASTY PEPPERY BEEF WITH TOMATO

Preparation Time: 15 minutes Cooking Time: 15minutes Servings: 8

Ingredients:

- 2 Tablespoons extra-virgin olive oil
- 1 large onion, chopped
- 1 large green bell pepper
- 4 garlic cloves, minced
- 1 jalapeño pepper, chopped
- 1 teaspoon dried thyme, crushed
- 1 teaspoon dried basil, crushed
- 2 Tablespoons red chili powder
- 1 Tablespoon ground cumin
- 1 teaspoon ground all spice
- 2 pounds grass-fed lean ground beef
- 3 cups fresh tomatoes, chopped finely
- 2 cups homemade chicken broth
- 1 cup water

Directions:

- In a large pan, warmth the oil over medium heat
- Sauté the onion and bell pepper for about 5-7 minutes.
- Add garlic, jalapeño pepper, herbs, spices and black pepper and sauté for about 1 minute.
- Then the beef and cook for about 4-5 minutes.
- Stir in the tomatoes and cook for about 2 minutes.
- Add the chicken broth and water and bring to a boil
- Reduce the heat to low and simmer, covered for about 25minutes and Serve hot.

62) GARLIC LAMB WITH KIDNEY BEANS

Preparation Time: 15 minutes Cooking Time: 30 minutes Servings: 6

Ingredients:

- 11/2 Tablespoons extra-virgin olive oil, divided
- 1 cup onion, chopped
- 6 large garlic cloves, minced
- 2 dried New Mexico chiles, stemmed, seeded and torn
- 3 dried ancho chiles, stemmed, seeded and torn
- 2 teaspoons dried oregano, crushed
- 11/2 teaspoons ground cumin
- 2 large plum tomatoes, chopped
- 2 cups homemade chicken broth
- 1 pound grass-fed lamb stew meat, trimmed and cubed
- Salt and ground black pepper, as required
- 15 ounces cooked kidney beans

Directions:

- In an oven-proof pan, heat 1 Tablespoon of oil over medium heat
- Sauté the onion for about 4-5 minutes.
- Add the garlic, both chiles and spices and sauté for about 1 minute.
- Then the tomatoes and broth and bring to a boil.
- Reduce the heat to medium-low and simmer, covered for about 10 minutes.
- Warmth the oven to 325 degrees F. Arrange a rack in the center of the oven.
- Detach the pan from heat and set aside to cool slightly.
- Transfer the Chile mixture into a blender and pulse until pureed.
- Return the puree in the same pan.
- Meanwhile, in another pan, warmth the remaining oil over medium-high heat
- Cook the lamb with salt and black pepper k for about 3-4 minutes.
- Transfer the cooked lamb in the pan with puree and stir to combine.
- Cover the pan and bake for about 30 minutes.
- Detach pan from the oven and place over medium-low heat.
- Simmer, uncovered for about 5 minutes.
- Stir in kidney beans and simmer for about 5 minutes.
- Serve hot.

63) SWEET AND SPICY ORANGE CHICKEN

Preparation Time: 10 minutes Cooking Time: 20 minutes Servings: 6

Ingredients:

- 3 garlic cloves, minced
- 1/2 cup fresh orange juice
- 1 Tablespoon apple cider vinegar
- 2 Tablespoons coconut amino
- 1/2 teaspoon orange blossom water
- 1/4 teaspoon ground ginger
- 1/4 teaspoon ground cinnamon
- Salt, as required
- 2 pounds grass-fed skinless, bone-in

Directions:

- For marinade, in a large bowl, place all ingredients except chicken and mix well.
- Add the chicken and coat with marinade generously.
- Cover the bowl of chicken and refrigerate for about 2 hours.
- Remove the chicken from bowl, reserving marinade.
- Heat a large nonstick wok, over medium-high heat
- Cook the chicken for about 5-6 minutes or until golden brown.
- Flip the side and cook for about 4 minutes.
- Add the reserved marinade and bring to a boil.
- Now, reduce the heat to medium-low heat and cook, covered for about 6-8 minutes or until sauce becomes thick.
- Serve hot.

64) HOMEMADE PINEAPPLE GRILLED CHICKEN

Preparation Time: 15 minutes Cooking Time: 20 minutes Servings: 4

Ingredients:

- 1 (1-inch) piece fresh ginger, minced
- 2 garlic cloves, minced
- 1 cup fresh pineapple juice
- 1/4 cup coconut amino
- 1/4 cup extra-virgin olive oil
- 1 teaspoon ground cinnamon
- 1 teaspoon ground cumin
- Salt, as required
- 4 grass-fed skinless, boneless chicken breasts

Directions:

- In a large Ziploc bag merge all ingredients and seal it.
- Shake the bag to coat the chicken with marinade well.
- Refrigerate to marinade for about 1 hour.
- Preheat the grill to medium-high heat. Grease the grill grate.
- Set the chicken breasts onto the grill and cook for about 10 minutes per side.
- Serve hot.

65) HOT AND SPICY PINEAPPLE COCONUT CHICKEN

Preparation Time: 20 minutes Cooking Time: 25 minutes Servings: 5

Ingredients:

- 1 Tablespoon extra-virgin olive oil
- 1 large onion, chopped
- 1 garlic clove, minced
- teaspoon fresh ginger, minced
- 2 grass-fed skinless, boneless chicken breasts, cubed
- 2 cups fresh pineapple, cubed
- 2 tomatoes, seeded

Ingredients:

- 1 medium red bell pepper
- 1 medium green bell pepper
- 1 medium orange bell pepper
- 2 Tablespoons coconut amino
- 1 Tablespoon apple cider vinegar
- Ground black pepper, as required

Directions:

- ❖ In a large skillet, heat oil over medium heat.
- ❖ Add onion and sauté for about 4-5 minutes.
- ❖ Add garlic and ginger and sauté for about 1 minute.
- ❖ Add chicken and cook for about 10 minutes or until browned from all sides.
- ❖ Add pineapple, tomatoes and bell peppers and cook for about 5-6 minutes or until vegetables become tender.
- ❖ Add the coconut amino, vinegar and pepper and cook for about 2-3 minutes.
- ❖ Serve hot.

66) NUTTY FRUITY CHICKEN ZUCCHINI NOODLES

Preparation Time: 15 minutes Cooking Time: 15 minutes Servings: 3

Ingredients:

- 2 zucchinis, spiralized with Blade C
- Salt, as required
- 11/2 teaspoons olive oil
- 1/2 teaspoon fresh ginger, minced
- 3/4 cup rhubarb, chopped
- 10 ounces grass-fed skinless, boneless chicken breasts, cubed
- 4 teaspoons raw honey

Ingredients:

- 1 teaspoon fresh lime zest, grated finely
- 1/4 cup fresh orange juice, divided
- 1 Tablespoon fresh lime juice
- 2 teaspoons fresh mint leaves, minced
- 1/2 cup fresh strawberries
- 2 Tablespoons almonds, toasted and slivered

Directions:

- ❖ Arrange a large strainer over the sink.
- ❖ 2Set the zucchini noodles in a strainer and sprinkle with a pinch of salt.
- ❖ Set aside to release the excess moisture.
- ❖ In a large skillet, warmth the oil over medium heat and cook the ginger and rhubarb for about 2-3 minutes.
- ❖ Stir in the chicken cubes and cook for about 4-5 minutes.
- ❖ Add the honey, lime zest, 1/4 cup of orange juice, lime juice and a pinch of salt and stir to combine.
- ❖ Now, set the heat to high and bring to a boil.
- ❖
- ❖ Now, reduce the heat to medium and simmer for about 4-5 minutes, stirring occasionally.
- ❖ Remove from the heat.
- ❖ Meanwhile, squeeze the moisture from zucchini and pat dry with paper towels.
- ❖ In a small bowl, place the remaining orange juice and mint and mix.
- ❖ Divide the zucchini noodles in serving plates and drizzle with mint mixture.
- ❖ 13. Place the chicken mixture, strawberries and almonds over zucchini noodles and gently stir to combine.
- ❖ 14. Serve immediately.

67) ROSEMARY PEPPER CHICKEN WITH BROCCOLI FLORETS

Preparation Time: 15 minutes | Cooking Time: 30 minutes | Servings: 6

Ingredients:

- 6 (6-ounce) grass-fed skinless, boneless chicken thighs
- 3 broccoli heads, cut into florets
- 4 garlic cloves, minced
- 1/4 cup extra-virgin olive oil
- 1 teaspoon dried oregano, crushed
- 1 teaspoon dried rosemary, crushed
- Salt and ground black pepper, as required

Directions:

- Set the oven to 375 degrees F. Grease a large baking dish.
- In a large bowl, merge all ingredients and toss to coat well.
- Set the broccoli florets and top with chicken breasts in a single layer.
- Bake for about 25 minutes.
- Serve hot.

68) APPLE GLAZED ROASTED TURKEY BREAST

Preparation Time: 20 minutes | Cooking Time: 30 minutes | Servings: 3

Ingredients:

For Turkey Rub:

- 1 (5-pound) whole, bone-in turkey breast
- 2 Tablespoons fresh thyme leaves, chopped
- 2 Tablespoons fresh rosemary, chopped
- 2 Tablespoons olive oil For Stuffing:
- 1 small onion, thinly sliced
- 1 apple, peeled and thinly sliced
- 1 pear, peeled and thinly sliced
- 1/4 cup dried cranberries

For Glaze:

- 2 cups fresh apple juice, divided
- 1 Tablespoon olive oil
- 1 Tablespoon brown mustard
- 1/2 Tablespoon coconut sugar

Directions:

- Warmth the oven to 325 degrees F. set a rack in a roasting pan.
- Arrange turkey breast into the prepared roasting pan, skin-side up.
- Use your fingers; gently loosen the skin from the meat
- Make deep pockets between the skin and meat.
- For rub: in a small bowl, merge together fresh herbs and oil.
- Rub half of herb mixture on the meat and then, spread the
- remaining paste evenly over the top of the skin.
- For stuffing: in a bowl, mix together all ingredients.
- Stuff each pocket with the stuffing mixture.
-
- 10. In the bottom of roasting pan, pour 1 cup of apple juice.
- 11. Roast for about 30 minutes
- (If skin becomes brown during roasting, then cover the pan with a piece of foil).
- 12. Meanwhile, for glaze: in a pan,
- 13. Add remaining apple juice, oil, mustard and brown sugar and bring to a boil.
- 14. Reduce the heat and simmer until thick glaze is formed.
- 15. In the last 5 minutes of cooking, coat turkey breast with glaze evenly.
- 16. Remove from oven and cut turkey into desired slices before serving.

69) SWEET AND SPICY ARROWROOT FLANK STEAK

Preparation Time: 15 minutes Cooking Time: 12 minutes Servings: 4

Ingredients:

- 2 Tablespoons arrowroot flour
- Salt and ground black pepper, as required
- 1 pound grass-fed flank steak, cut into 1/4-inch thick slices
- 1/2 cup plus 1 Tablespoon coconut oil, divided
- 2 garlic cloves, minced
- 1 teaspoon ground ginger
- Pinch of red pepper flakes, crushed
- 1/3 cup raw honey
- 1/2 cup homemade beef broth
- 1/2 cup coconut amino
- 3 scallions, chopped

Directions:

- ❖ In a bowl, attach the arrowroot flour, salt and black pepper and mix well.
- ❖ Coat the beef slices with arrowroot flour mixture evenly.
- ❖ Shake off the excess arrowroot flour mixture and set aside for about 10-15 minutes.
- ❖ For sauce: in a pan, melt 1 Tablespoon of coconut oil over medium heat
- ❖ Sauté the garlic, ginger powder and red pepper flakes for about 1 minute.
- ❖ Add the honey, broth and coconut amino and stir to combine well.
- ❖ Remove from the heat and set aside.
- ❖ 8. In a large skillet, dissolve the remaining coconut oil over medium heat
- ❖ 9. Stir fry the beef for about 2-3 minutes.
- ❖ 10. Remove the oil from skillet and stir fry for about 1 minute.
- ❖ 11. Stir in the honey sauce and cook for about 3 minutes.
- ❖ 12. Stir in the scallion and cook for about 1 minute more.
- ❖ 13. Serve hot.

70) STUFFED PEPPERS

Preparation Time: 10 minutes Cooking Time: 25 minutes Servings: 4

Ingredients:

- 12 ounces grass-fed lean ground beef
- 4 green bell peppers
- 1 cup cauliflower, grated
- 1/4 cup sundried tomato
- 1 medium onion, minced
- 4 cloves garlic, minced
- 2 cups tomato puree
- 1 teaspoon oregano
- 1/2 teaspoon cinnamon
- 1 teaspoon salt
- 1 teaspoon black pepper
- Olive oil

Directions:

- ❖ 1. Set 2 tablespoons olive oil in skillet; add onion and garlic and sauté for one minute.
- ❖ 2. Place half of the mixture into a slow cooker, along with tomato puree, and mix.
- ❖ 3. Add beef to skillet, brown, and drain.
- ❖ 4. Mix beef and onion with grated cauliflower and sundried tomatoes, salt, black pepper, cinnamon, and oregano.
- ❖ 5. Slice the tops off the peppers, detach seeds, and stuff peppers with cauliflower mixture.
- ❖ 6. Place peppers in the slow cooker and cook on low for 7 hours.

71) HEARTY WINTER QUINOA SOUP

Preparation Time: 10 minutes Cooking Time: 25 minutes Servings: 4

Ingredients:

- 2 tablespoons olive oil
- 1 onion, chopped
- 2 carrots, peeled and chopped
- 1 parsnip, chopped
- 1 celery stalk, chopped
- 1 cup yellow squash, chopped
- 4 garlic cloves, pressed or minced
- 4 cups roasted vegetable broth
- 2 medium tomatoes, crushed
- 1 cup quinoa
- Sea salt and ground black pepper, to taste
- 1 bay laurel
- 2 cup Swiss chard, tough ribs removed and torn into pieces
- 2 tablespoons Italian parsley, chopped

Directions:

- ❖ In a heavy-bottomed pot, heat the olive over medium-high heat
- ❖ Now, sauté the onion, carrot, parsnip, celery and yellow squash for about 3 minutes
- ❖ (Or until the vegetables are just tender.
- ❖ Add in the garlic and continue to sauté for 1 minute or until aromatic.
- ❖ Then, stir in the vegetable broth, tomatoes, quinoa, salt, pepper
- ❖ Join also bay laurel; bring to a boil
- ❖ Immediately reduce the heat to a simmer and let it cook for 13 minutes.
- ❖ Fold in the Swiss chard; continue to simmer until the chard wilts.
- ❖ Ladle into individual bowls and serve garnished with the fresh parsley

72) GREEN LENTIL SALAD

Preparation Time: 10 minutes Cooking Time: 20 minutes Servings: 5

Ingredients:

- 1 ½ cups green lentils, rinsed
- 2 cups arugula
- 2 cups Romaine lettuce, torn into pieces
- 1 cup baby spinach
- 1/4 cup fresh basil, chopped
- 1/2 cup shallots, chopped
- 2 garlic cloves, finely chopped
- 1/4 cup oil-packed sun-dried tomatoes, rinsed and chopped
- 5 tablespoons extra-virgin olive oil
- 3 tablespoons fresh lemon juice
- Sea salt and ground black pepper, to taste

Directions:

- ❖ In a large-sized saucepan, bring 4 ½ cups of the water and red lentils to a boil.
- ❖ Immediately turn the heat to a simmer
- ❖ Continue to cook your lentils for a further 15 to 17 minutes or until they've softened but not mushy.
- ❖ Drain and let it cool completely. Transfer the lentils to a salad bowl
- ❖ Toss the lentils with the remaining Ingredients until well combined.
- ❖ Serve chilled or at room temperature

73) ACORN SQUASH, CHICKPEA AND COUSCOUS SOUP

Preparation Time: 10 minutes Cooking Time: 20 minutes Servings: 4

Ingredients:

- 2 tablespoons olive oil
- 1 shallot, chopped
- 1 carrot, trimmed and chopped
- 2 cups acorn squash, chopped
- 1 stalk celery, chopped
- 1 teaspoon garlic, finely chopped
- 1 teaspoon dried rosemary, chopped
- 1 teaspoon dried thyme, chopped
- 2 cups cream of onion soup
- 2 cups water
- 1 cup dry couscous
- Sea salt and ground black pepper, to taste
- 1/2 teaspoon red pepper flakes
- 6 ounces canned chickpeas, drained
- 2 tablespoons fresh lemon juice

Directions:

- ❖ In a heavy-bottomed pot, heat the olive over medium-high heat.
- ❖ Now, sauté the shallot, carrot, acorn squash and celery for about 3 minutes
- ❖ (Or until the vegetables are just tender)
- ❖ Add in the garlic, rosemary and thyme and continue to sauté for 1 minute or until aromatic.
- ❖ Then, stir in the soup, water, couscous, salt, black pepper and red pepper flakes
- ❖ Bring to a boil. Immediately reduce the heat to a simmer and let it cook for 12 minutes.
- ❖ Fold in the canned chickpeas; continue to simmer until heated through or about 5 minutes more.
- ❖ Ladle into individual bowls and drizzle with the lemon juice over the top.

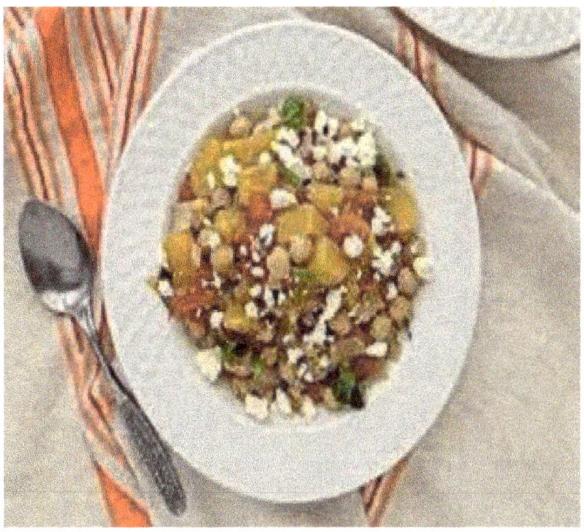

74) CABBAGE SOUP WITH GARLIC CROSTINI

Preparation Time: 10 minutes Cooking Time: 1 hours Servings: 4

Ingredients:

Soup:

- 2 tablespoons olive oil
- 1 medium leek, chopped 1 cup turnip, chopped
- 1 parsnip, chopped
- 1 carrot, chopped
- 2 cups cabbage, shredded
- 2 garlic cloves, finely chopped
- 4 cups vegetable broth
- 2 bay leaves

Ingredients:

Crostini:

- Sea salt and ground black pepper, to taste
- 1/4 teaspoon cumin seeds
- 1/2 teaspoon mustard seeds
- 1 teaspoon dried basil
- 2 tomatoes, pureed
- 8 slices of baguette
- 2 heads garlic
- 4 tablespoons extra-virgin olive oil

Directions:

- ❖ In a soup pot, heat 2 tablespoons of the olive over medium-high heat.
- ❖ Now, sauté the leek, turnip, parsnip and carrot for about 4 minutes or until the vegetables are crisp-tender.
- ❖ Add in the garlic and cabbage and continue to sauté for 1 minute or until aromatic.
- ❖ Then, stir in the vegetable broth, bay leaves, salt, black pepper
- ❖ Add cumin seeds, mustard seeds, dried basil and pureed tomatoes
- ❖ Bring to a boil. Immediately reduce the heat to a simmer and let it cook for about 20 minutes.
- ❖ Meanwhile, preheat your oven to 375 degrees F
- ❖ Now, roast the garlic and baguette slices for about 15 minutes. Remove the crostini from the oven.
- ❖ Continue baking the garlic for 45 minutes more or until very tender
- ❖ Allow the garlic to cool.
- ❖ Now, cut each head of the garlic using a sharp serrated knife in order to separate all the cloves.
- ❖ Squeeze the roasted garlic cloves out of their skins
- ❖ Mash the garlic pulp with 4 tablespoons of the extra-virgin olive oil.
- ❖ Spread the roasted garlic mixture evenly on the tops of the crostini
- ❖ Serve with the warm soup

75) CREAM OF GREEN BEAN SOUP

Preparation Time: 10 minutes Cooking Time: 35 minutes Servings: 4

Ingredients:

- 1 tablespoon sesame oil
- 1 onion, chopped
- 1 green pepper, seeded and chopped
- 2 russet potatoes, peeled and diced
- 2 garlic cloves, chopped
- 4 cups vegetable broth
- 1-pound green beans, trimmed
- Sea salt and ground black pepper, to season
- 1 cup full-fat coconut milk

Directions:

- ❖ In a heavy-bottomed pot, heat the sesame over medium-high heat.
- ❖ Now, sauté the onion, peppers and potatoes for about 5 minutes, stirring periodically.
- ❖ Add in the garlic and continue sautéing for 1 minute or until fragrant.
- ❖ Then, stir in the vegetable broth, green beans, salt and black pepper; bring to a boil. Immediately reduce the heat to a simmer and let it cook for 20 minutes.
- ❖ Puree the green bean mixture using an immersion blender until creamy and uniform.
- ❖ Return the pureed mixture to the pot. Fold in the coconut milk and continue to simmer until heated through or about 5 minutes longer.
- ❖ Ladle into individual bowls and serve hot.

76) TRADITIONAL FRENCH ONION SOUP

Preparation Time: 10 minutes Cooking Time: 1 hour 30 minutes Servings: 4

Ingredients:

- 2 tablespoons olive oil
- 2 large yellow onions, thinly sliced
- 2 thyme sprigs, chopped
- 2 rosemary sprigs, chopped
- 2 teaspoons balsamic vinegar
- 4 cups vegetable stock
- Sea salt and ground black pepper, to taste

Directions:

- ❖ In a or Dutch oven, heat the olive oil over a moderate heat.
- ❖ Now, cook the onions with thyme, rosemary and 1 teaspoon of the sea salt for about 2 minutes.
- ❖ Turn the heat to medium-low and continue cooking until the onions caramelize or about 50 minutes.
- ❖ Add in the balsamic vinegar and continue to cook for a further 15 more.
- ❖ Then in the stock, salt and black pepper and continue simmering for 20 to 25 minutes.
- ❖ Serve with toasted bread and enjoy!

77) ROASTED CARROT SOUP

Preparation Time: 10 minutes   Cooking Time: 50 minutes   Servings: 4

Ingredients:

- 1 ½ pounds carrots
- 4 tablespoons olive oil
- 1 yellow onion, chopped
- 2 cloves garlic, minced
- 1/3 teaspoon ground cumin
- Sea salt and white pepper, to taste
- 1/2 teaspoon turmeric powder
- 4 cups vegetable stock
- 2 teaspoons lemon juice
- 2 tablespoons fresh cilantro, roughly chopped

Directions:

- ❖ Start by preheating your oven to 400 degrees F.
- ❖ Place the carrots on a large parchment-lined baking sheet
- ❖ Toss the carrots with 2 tablespoons of the olive oil.
- ❖ Roast the carrots for about 35 minutes or until they've softened.
- ❖ In a heavy-bottomed pot, heat the remaining 2 tablespoons of the olive oil
- ❖ Now, sauté the onion and garlic for about 3 minutes or until aromatic.
- ❖ Add in the cumin, salt, pepper, turmeric, vegetable stock and roasted carrots
- ❖ Continue to simmer for 12 minutes more.
- ❖ Puree your soup with an immersion blender
- ❖ Drizzle lemon juice over your soup and serve garnished with fresh cilantro leaves

78) ITALIAN PENNE PASTA SALAD

Preparation Time: 10 minutes   Cooking Time: 15 minutes   Servings: 3

Ingredients:

- 9 ounces penne pasta
- 9 ounces canned Cannellini bean, drained
- 1 small onion, thinly sliced
- 1/3 cup Niçoise olives, pitted and sliced
- 2 Italian peppers, sliced
- 1 cup cherry tomatoes, halved
- 3 cups arugula

Dressing:

- 3 tablespoons extra-virgin olive oil
- 1 teaspoon lemon zest
- 1 teaspoon garlic, minced
- 3 tablespoons balsamic vinegar
- 1 teaspoon Italian herb mix
- Sea salt and ground black pepper, to taste

Directions:

- ❖ Cook the penne pasta according to the package Directions
- ❖ Drain and rinse the pasta. Let it cool completely and then, transfer it to a salad bowl.
- ❖ Then, add the beans, onion, olives, peppers, tomatoes and arugula to the salad bowl.
- ❖
- ❖
- ❖ Mix all the dressing Ingredients until everything is well incorporated.
- ❖ Dress your salad and serve well-chilled

79) ARUGULA WITH FRUITS AND NUTS

Preparation Time: 10 minutes | Cooking Time: 0 minutes | Servings: 1

Ingredients:

- ½ cup arugula
- ½ peach
- ½ red onion
- ¼ cup blueberries
- 5 walnuts, chopped
- 1 tbsp. extra-virgin olive oil
- 2 tbsp. red wine vinegar
- 1 spring of fresh basil

Directions:

- ❖ Halve the peach and remove the seed. Heat a grill pan and grill it briefly on both sides
- ❖ Cut the red onion into thin half-rings. Roughly chop the pecans.
- ❖ Heat a pan and roast the pecans in it until they are fragrant.
- ❖ Place the arugula on a plate and spread peaches, red onions, blueberries, and roasted pecans over it.
- ❖ Put all the ingredients for the dressing in a food processor and mix to an even dressing
- ❖ Drizzle the dressing over the salad.

80) BROCCOLI SALAD

Preparation Time: 25 minutes | Cooking Time: 0 minutes | Servings: 2

Ingredients:

- 1 head of broccoli
- 1/2 red onion
- 2 carrots, grated
- ¼ cup red grapes
- 2 1/2 tbsp. Coconut yogurt
- 1 tbsp. Water
- 1 tsp. mustard
- 1 pinch salt

Directions:

- ❖ Cut the broccoli into florets and cook for 8 minutes.
- ❖ Cut the red onion into thin half-rings. Halve the grapes
- ❖ Mix coconut yogurt, water, and mustard with a pinch of salt to make the dressing.
- ❖ Drain the broccoli and rinse with ice-cold water to stop the cooking process.
- ❖ Mix the broccoli with the carrot, onion, and red grapes in a bowl
- ❖ Serve the dressing separately on the side.

DESSERT RECIPES

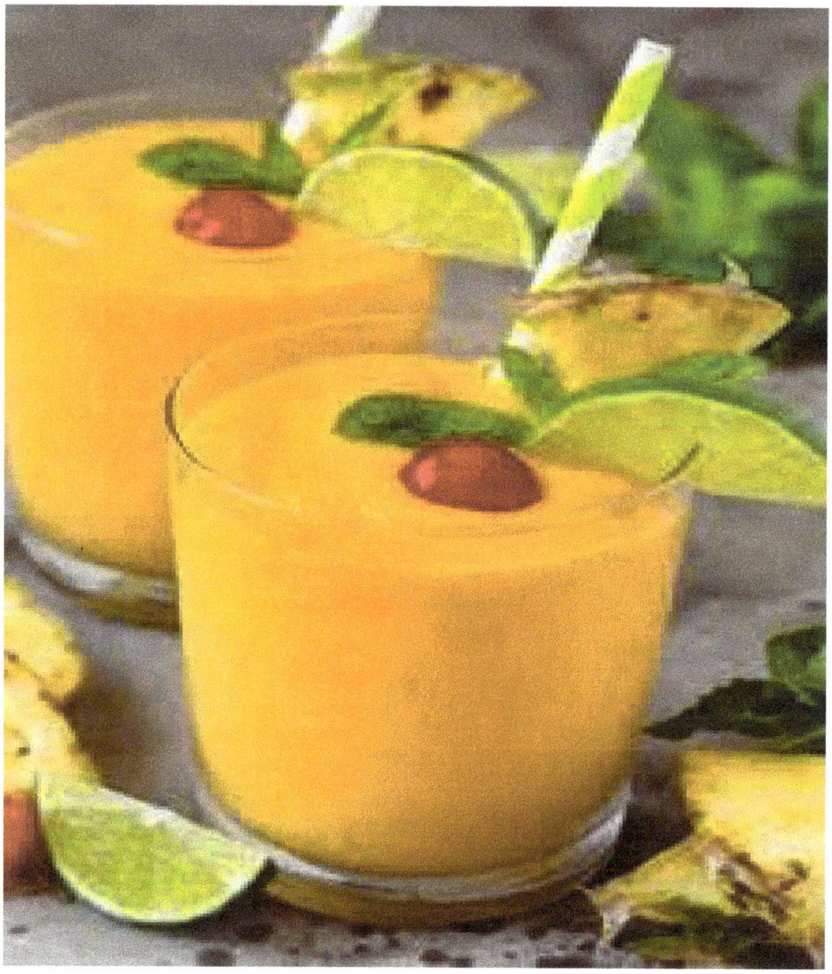

81) TROPICAL SMOOTHIE

Preparation Time: 5 minutes Cooking Time: 5 minutes Servings: 1

Ingredients:

- 1 banana
- 1 pineapple
- 1 cup mango
- 1 cup almond milk

Directions:

- ❖ In a blender merge all ingredients and blend until smooth
- ❖ Pour smoothie in a glass and serve

82) BERRY SMOOTHIE

Preparation Time: 5 minutes Cooking Time: 5 minutes Servings: 1

Ingredients:

- 1 banana
- 4 cups pineapple juice
- 1 cup ice
- 4 oz. blueberries
- 4 oz. blackberries
- 1 tablespoon honey

Directions:

- ❖ In a blender merge all ingredients and blend until smooth
- ❖ Pour smoothie in a glass and serve

83) CITRUS SMOOTHIE

Preparation Time: 5 minutes Cooking Time: 5 minutes Servings: 1

Ingredients:

- 1 cup carrot juice 1 banana
- 1 cup pineapple juice 1 cup ice

Directions:

- ❖ In a blender merge all ingredients and blend until smooth
- ❖ Pour smoothie in a glass and serve

84) POMEGRANATE SMOOTHIE

Preparation Time: 5 minutes   Cooking Time: 5 minutes   Servings: 1

Ingredients:

- 1 cup pomegranate juice
- 1 cup yogurt
- 1 cup berries

Ingredients:

- 1 cup ice
- 1 cinnamon

Directions:

- In a blender merge all ingredients and blend until smooth
- Pour smoothie in a glass and serve

85) PEANUT BUTTER SMOOTHIE

Preparation Time: 5 minutes   Cooking Time: 5 minutes   Servings: 1

Ingredients:

- 1 banana
- 1 cup milk

Ingredients:

- 2 tablespoons peanut butter
- 1 cup ice

Directions:

- ❖ In a blender merge all ingredients and blend until smooth
- ❖ Pour smoothie in a glass and serve

86) MANGO SMOOTHIE

Preparation Time: 5 minutes   Cooking Time: 5 minutes   Servings: 1

Ingredients:

- 1 cup orange juice
- 1/4 cup vanilla yogurt
- 1 cup mango

Ingredients:

- 1 carrot
- 1 cup Ice

Directions:

- ❖ In a blender merge all ingredients and blend until smooth
- ❖ Pour smoothie in a glass and serve

87) GREEN CITRUS SMOOTHIE

Preparation Time: 10 minutes | Cooking Time: 0 minutes | Servings: 2

Ingredients:

- 1 cup chopped watercress
- 1 large grapefruit, peeled
- 2 medium oranges, peeled
- 1 medium banana, peeled
- 1 cup water, divided

Directions:

- Place watercress, grapefruit, oranges, banana, and 1/2 cup water in a blender and blend until thoroughly combined.
- Add remaining water while blending until desired texture is achieved.

88) CHERRY PEAR SMOOTHIE

Preparation Time: 10 minutes | Cooking Time: 0 minutes | Servings: 2

Ingredients:

- 1 cup chopped iceberg lettuce
- 2 medium pears, cored
- 1medium banana, peeled
- 1/2 cup pitted cherries
- 1/2 teaspoon vanilla bean pulp
- 2 cups unsweetened vanilla almond milk, divided

Directions:

- Place lettuce, pears, banana, cherries, vanilla bean pulp, and 1 cup almond milk in a blender and blend until thoroughly combined
- Add remaining almond milk while blending until desired texture is achieved

89) APPLE PEACH SMOOTHIE

Preparation Time: 10 minutes | Cooking Time: 0 minutes | Servings: 2

Ingredients:

- 2 tablespoons rolled oats
- 1 cup chopped watercress
- 2 medium peaches, pitted
- 2 medium apples, cored and peeled
- 2 cups unsweetened vanilla almond milk, divided

Directions:

- Place oats, watercress, peaches, apples, and 1 cup almond milk in a blender and blend until thoroughly combined.
- Add remaining almond milk while blending until desired texture is achieved.

90) ZUCCHINI APPLE SMOOTHIE

Preparation Time: 10 minutes   Cooking Time: 0 minutes   Servings: 2

Ingredients:

- 1 cup spinach
- 1 medium zucchini, chopped
- 3 medium carrots, peeled and chopped
- 2 medium apples, cored and peeled
- 2 cups water, divided

Directions:

❖ Place spinach, zucchini, carrots, apples, and 1 cup water in a blender and blend until thoroughly combined.

❖ Add remaining water while blending until desired texture is achieved.

91) CHOCOLATE CHIP COOKIES

Preparation Time: 20 minutes   Cooking Time: 13 minutes   Servings: 4

Ingredients:

- 1 oz paleo chocolate chips
- 1 egg, beaten
- 1 cup almond flour
- 2 tablespoons flax meal
- 1 teaspoon baking powder
- 3 tablespoons almond butter
- 1 teaspoon raw honey

Directions:

❖ In the mixing bowl mix up egg, almond flour, flax meal, baking powder, raw honey, and almond butter.

❖ Stir the mixture with the help of the spoon and add chocolate chips.

❖ Knead the non-sticky dough.

❖ Make the big ball from the dough and cut it on small pieces.

❖ Roll the small balls from the dough pieces.

❖ Line the baking tray with baking paper.

❖ Press the dough balls gently and arrange in the baking tray.

❖ Bake the cooked for 13 minutes at 360F.

❖ Then cool the cooked cookies well and store them in the glass jar.

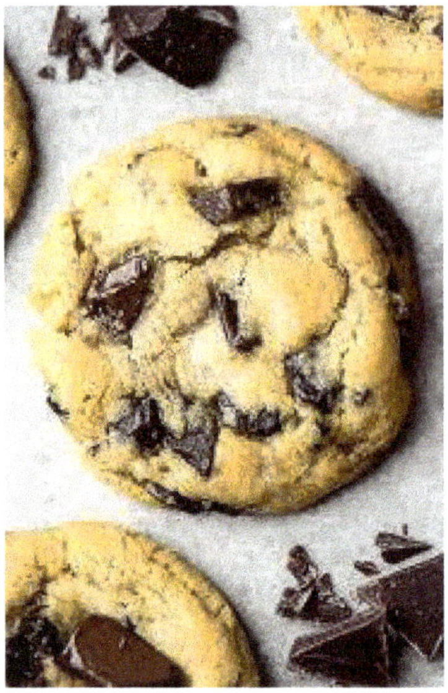

92) LEMON BREAD

Preparation Time: 20 minutes | Cooking Time: 25 minutes | Servings: 6

Ingredients:

- 1 cup almond flour
- ½ cup chestnut flour
- ¼ cup lemon juice
- 2 teaspoons lemon zest, grated
- 5 eggs, beaten
- ¼ cup coconut cream
- 2 teaspoons baking powder
- 2 tablespoons coconut oil, melted
- 1 tablespoon vanilla extract
- 1 tablespoon raw honey
- ¼ teaspoon ground cinnamon

Directions:

- Preheat the oven to 360F.
- Line the loaf mold with the baking paper.
- After this, in the mixing bowl mix up chestnuts, lemon juice, lemon zest, eggs, coconut cream, baking powder, coconut oil, vanilla extract, raw honey, and ground cinnamon.
- Stir the mixture with the help of the spoon until you get a smooth batter.
- Then pour it in the prepared loaf mold.
- Flatten the surface of the batter and transfer it in the preheated oven.
- Bake the lemon bread for 25 minutes.
- Then switch off the oven and let the bread stay there for 10 minutes more.

93) SWEET SMOOTHIE BOWL

Preparation Time: 15 minutes | Cooking Time: 0 minutes | Servings: 4

Ingredients:

- 2 cups cherries, frozen
- 2 bananas, peeled, frozen
- 1 tablespoon coconut shred
- 1 cup organic almond milk
- 4 strawberries, sliced

Directions:

- Put cherries, bananas, and almond milk in the blender.
- Blend the mixture until it is smooth.
- Then transfer the smoothie mixture in the serving bowls.
- Top them with coconut shred and sliced strawberries.

94) MANGO SALAD

Preparation Time: 10 minutes | Cooking Time: 0 minutes | Servings: 4

Ingredients:

- 1 mango, peeled, chopped
- 1 banana, chopped
- 1 kiwi, peeled, chopped
- 2 tablespoons organic almond milk
- 1 teaspoon raw honey
- 1 tablespoon almonds, chopped

Directions:

- In the big bowl mix up chopped mango, kiwi, and almonds.
- Then add bananas and shake the salad well.
- After this, sprinkle the salad with almond milk and honey.
- Gently stir the cooked dessert before serving.

95) APRICOT AND HAZELNUT BARS

Preparation Time: 15 minutes | Cooking Time: 17 minutes | Servings: 4

Ingredients:

- 2 apricots, chopped
- 4 oz hazelnuts, chopped
- 1 cup cassava flour
- 2 eggs, beaten
- 1 tablespoon coconut sugar
- ¼ cup organic almond milk
- 1 tablespoon almond butter

Directions:

- In the mixing bowl mix up chopped hazelnuts, cassava flour, eggs, coconut sugar, almond milk, and almond butter.
- When the mixture is smooth, add chopped apricots and stir it.
- After this, line the baking tray with the baking paper and pour the apricot mixture inside. Flatten it if needed.
- Preheat the oven to 365F.
- Put the tray with the apricot batter in the oven and cook for 17 minutes.
- Then cool the meal and cut it on the serving bars.

96) WALNUT MUFFINS

Preparation Time: 15 minutes | Cooking Time: 12 minutes | Servings: 6

Ingredients:

- ½ cup tapioca flour
- ½ cup almond flour
- ½ cup walnuts, grinded
- 3 tablespoons raw honey
- 3 eggs, beaten
- 1 teaspoon baking powder
- 1 teaspoon vanilla extract
- 2 tablespoons coconut oil

Directions:

- In the mixing bowl mix up tapioca flour, almond flour, and walnuts,
- Then add eggs, honey, baking powder, vanilla extract, and coconut oil.
- Stir the mixture until smooth.
- Then preheat the oven to 360F.
- Pour the walnut muffin batter in the molds (fill ½ part of every muffin mold) and transfer them in the oven.
- Bake the muffins for 12 minutes.

97) STRAWBERRIES IN COCONUT CREAM

Preparation Time: 15 minutes | Cooking Time: 0 minutes | Servings: 2

Ingredients:

- 1 cup strawberries
- ½ cup coconut cream
- 1 tablespoon coconut sugar
- 1 teaspoon vanilla extract
- ¼ teaspoon dried mint

Directions:

- In the mixing bowl mix up coconut cream, coconut sugar, vanilla extract, and dried mint.
- Whisk the mixture until it is smooth and lightly fluffy.
- Then chop the strawberries roughly and put in the serving bowls.
- Top the berries with fluffy coconut cream mixture.

98) BERRIES AND PANCAKE SKEWERS

Preparation Time: 10 minutes | Cooking Time: 10 minutes | Servings: 2

Ingredients:

- ¼ cup strawberries
- ½ cup arrowroot flour
- 1 teaspoon baking powder
- 1 teaspoon raw honey
- 3 eggs, beaten
- 1 teaspoon olive oil

Directions:

- In the mixing bowl mix up arrowroot flour, baking powder, and eggs.
- Whisk the mixture well.
- Then pour olive oil in the skillet and heat it up.
- Pour the small amount of the arrowroot flour dough in the skillet to make the small pancakes.
- Fry them for 1 minute from each side.
- Then string the strawberries and pancakes on the skewers one-by-one.

99) CARAMEL APPLES

Preparation Time: 10 minutes | Cooking Time: 10 minutes | Servings: 4

Ingredients:

- 4 teaspoons coconut sugar
- 2 pecans, chopped
- 1 teaspoon almonds, chopped
- 1 tablespoon almond butter
- ¼ teaspoon ground clove
- 4 apples

Directions:

- Core the apples and chop them roughly.
- Then heat up the skillet well.
- Put the almond butter in the hot skillet and melt it.
- Add coconut sugar, almonds, and ground clove.
- Stir the mixture well and preheat it on low heat until sugar is dissolved.
- Then add chopped apples and coat them well in the hot sugar mixture (caramel).
- Transfer the apples in the serving plates.

100) CARROT MUFFINS

Preparation Time: 15 minutes Cooking Time: 14 minutes Servings: 4

Ingredients:

- ¼ cup carrot, grated
- 1 teaspoon vanilla extract
- 1 cup coconut flour
- 1 teaspoon baking powder
- 1 teaspoon lemon juice
- 1 teaspoon ground nutmeg
- 2 tablespoons coconut oil, melted
- 1 tablespoon coconut sugar
- 4 eggs, beaten

Directions:

- In the mixing bowl mix up vanilla extract, coconut flour, baking powder, lemon juice, ground nutmeg, coconut oil, and coconut sugar.
- Then add eggs and stir the mixture until it is smooth.
- After this, add a grated carrot and stir it until smooth again.
- Preheat the oven to 355F.
- Fill ½ part of every muffin mold with carrot muffin batter and bake them in the oven for 14 minutes.
- Cool the muffins well and remove them from the molds.

CPSIA information can be obtained
at www.ICGtesting.com
Printed in the USA
LVHW061659010621
689062LV00008B/398

9 781803 014302